EASY BREAD MACHINE

INTRODUCTION

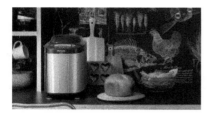

Bread making machine, also called a bread producer, is a locally situated apparatus that changes uncooked fixings into bread. It is comprised of a pot for bread (or "tin,") with at least one inherent oars at the base, present in the focal point of a little specific reason broiler. This little broiler is generally worked by means of a control board through a straightforward in-constructed PC using the information settings. Some bread machines have assorted cycles for different types of mixture along with white bread, entire grain, European-style (at times called"French"), and batter just (for pizza batter and framed portions prepared in a customary broiler). Many likewise have a clock to empower the bread machine to work without the administrator's participation, and some top of the line models permit the client to program a redid period.

To prepare bread, fixings are estimated in a predefined request into the bread container (generally first fluids, with strong fixings layered on top), and afterward the skillet is placed in the bread creator. The request for fixings is significant on the grounds that contact with water triggers the moment yeast utilized in bread producers, so the yeast and water must be kept separate until the program starts.
It takes the machine a few hours to make a bread portion. The items are refreshed first and brought to an ideal temperature. Mix with an oar, and the fixings are then formed into flour. Utilize ideal temperature guideline, and the mixture is then affirmed and afterward cooked.

When the bread has been heated, the bread creator eliminates the dish. Then leaving a slight indentation from the rod to which the paddle is connected. The completed portion's shape is regularly viewed as extraordinary. Many beginning bread machines fabricate an in an upward direction skewed towards, square, or barrel shaped portion that is fundamentally unique from business bread; notwithstanding, later units commonly have a more regular level skillet. Some bread machines utilize two oars to frame two lb. portion in standard square shape shape.

Bread machine plans are frequently a lot more modest than normal bread plans. Some of the time normalized in view of the machine's dish limit, the most famous in the US market is 1.5 lb./700 g units. Most plans are composed for that limit; in any case, two lb./900 g units are normal. There are arranged bread blends, exceptionally made for bread creators, containing preestimated fixings and flour and yeast, flavorings, and now and then batter conditioners.

Bread producers are likewise fitted with a clock for testing when breadproduction begins. For instance, this permits them to be stacked around evening time Notwithstanding just start baking in the first part of the day to create a newly heated bread for breakfast. They may likewise be set distinctly for making batter, for instance, for making pizza. Aside from bread, some can likewise be set to make different things like jam, pasta mixture, and Japanese rice cake. A portion of the new advancements in the office of the machine incorporates consequently adding nut. It additionally contains organic product from a plate during the massaging system. Bread creators ordinarily take somewhere in the range of three and four hours to heat a portion. However, later "speedy prepare" modes have become standard augmentations, a significant number of which can create a portion in under an hour.

CHAPTER 1:

Baking Process Made Easy

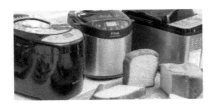

Bread is a heated food that can be set up from different sorts of player. The combination is usually made of flour and water. The sizes and sorts of flour and the various trimmings change, as do the laying methods. From the start bread was quite possibly the most fundamental food, just as perhaps the most settled fake. Surely, individuals have been making bread since the start of horticulture.

Bread is ordinarily organized from a wheat flour combination, which is made with yeast and allowed to rise. Ordinarily, people heat bread on the oven. Regardless, a consistently expanding number of people go to the phenomenal bread machines to plan crispbread at home.

What is a Bread Machine?
A bread machine is a kitchen apparatus for warming bread. The device is a digging tool or bread tin, made in the spatulas, which is situated in the focal point of a little multifunctional unique mesh.

How is Bread Machine Made?
This machine is basically a moderate electric apparatus that holds a lone, tremendous bread tin inside. The actual tin is to some degree unprecedented it has a center at the base that is related with an electric motor underneath. A little metal paddle is affixed to the turn at the foundation of the tin. The paddle is liable for controlling the blend. A waterproof seal gets the center point itself. We ought to explore all of the bread machine parts in detail:

-

The top over the bread producer comes either with the survey window or without it

The control board is likewise situated on the highest point of the bread machine with the end goal of comfort

.

In the focal point of the top, there is a steam vent that depletes the steam during the heating procedure. A portion of the bread creators likewise have an air vent on the gadget for air to come inside the tin for the mixture to rise

Benefits of a Bread Machine

.

You can appreciate the crisply prepared handcrafted bread. Most bread creators additionally include a clockwork, which permits you to set the preparing cycle at a specific time. This capacity is extremely valuable when you need to have sweltering bread toward the beginning of the day for breakfast.

.

You can control what you eat. By preparing bread at home, you can really control what parts are coming into your portion. This choice is extremely valuable for individuals with sensitivities or for those who attempt to control the admission of a fixings' portion.

.

It is simple. A few people believe that preparing bread at home is chaotic, and by and large, it is a hard procedure. In any case, preparing bread with a bread machine is a breeze. You simply pick the ideal choice and unwind - all the blending rising and heating

process is happening inside the bread maker, making it a zero turmoil process!
It sets aside your huge amounts of cash in the long haul. If you imagine that purchasing bread at a store is modest, you may be mixed up. It turns out that in the long haul, preparing bread at home will set aside your cash, particularly in the event that you have some dietary limitations.

.

Incredible taste and quality, you have to acknowledge it – nothing beats the quality and taste of a crisp heap of bread. Since you are the person who is making bread, you can ensure that you utilize just the fixings that are new and of a high caliber. Homemade bread consistently beats locally acquired bread as far as taste and quality.

How Does Bread Machine Work?

To start with, you put the employing paddle inside the tin. Right when the tin is out of the machine, you can check the trimmings and weight them into the tin.

Some time later, you basically need to put the skillet inside the oven (machine), pick the program you wish through the electronic load up, and close the top. Here the bread maker charm dominates!

One of the most compelling things the bread machine will do is working the hitter - you will hear the sounds. If your bread maker goes with the see window, you can watch the whole method of planning which is very interesting.

After the rubbing stage, all that will go quiet for a surprisingly long time - the rising stage comes. The machine permits the combination to batter and rise. By then, there will be one demonstrating.

Although the commonplace machines go with equation books that give you different fascinating moved bread plans.
more round of controlling and a time of

bread making process is modified, most

Bread Machine Cycles

Bread machines are a phenomenal kitchen assistant to own.

These little reduced miracles have numerous choices and settings for baking a variety of bread astonishingly. When you come out as comfortable with your bread machine's settings, the opportunity to make and examination is endless.

It is crucial for realize what each setting on your machine can convey, making it more clear which capacity to utilize when baking your portion. Being good friends with your bread machine will permit you to make flavorsome bread, making you wish you had bought the machine sooner!

Bread machines can come in two distinct assortments. A few brands hold explicit settings that you can't change, so it is shrewd to adhere to the guidance manual when making diverse bread styles to see which setting will be great, while some bread machines accompany fundamental settings with times and programming that you can modify. For example, in the event that you notice that the bread didn't ascend as you expected, you can expand the rising time. By permitting you to change a portion of the settings to suit your requirements, you can make the ideal portion of bread.

Now, let me comprehend the different cycles and settings you can find on your bread machine.

Basic

This is otherwise called essential bread, fundamental wheat, and essential mode, white or standard bread. This setting is most normally utilized for all reasons. The cycle goes on for up to three to four hours, in view of your machine, and is utilized for entire wheat or entire grain bread and white bread that are comprised of in excess of 50% bread flour. You can likewise utilize this cycle rather than a French bread cycle or then again in the event that your machine doesn't have a French bread cycle. In this essential cycle, there is now and then the choice for "speedy" or "quick." Or your machine can have the choices in a different cycle. On a significant number of the fresher models, there's an inbuilt ready that goes off when you really want to add any additional fixings, like raisins or nuts.

Sweet Bread

This cycle makes batters with higher sugar and Fat: content to rise more slow than expected. This Sweet Bread cycle has a more drawn out ascent time and a diminished baking temperature, pretty much 250 °F. This is on the grounds that the outside layer of the sweet bread will brown quicker. The inbuilt indicator in this cycle beeps when it's time to add the extra ingredients to the mix such as chopped glacéed fruit or nuts. Additionally, numerous sweetbreads are blended, molded in the batter cycle, and prepared in the home oven.

Fruit and Nut

This cycle is otherwise called the Raisin Mode or Mix Bread cycle. This setting is utilized when nuts, chocolate chips, seeds, or dried natural products are added to the mixture. With this strategy, the additional fixings are not overmixed or totally mixed during the outrageous speed of the edge activity during the massaging period of the cycle. Large numbers of the fresher models have a discernible caution inbuilt as a feature of the essential and entire wheat cycles, rather than worked in a different cycle. At the point when the alarm sounds, the time has come to open the cover and add the additional items. But if your machine doesn't have this cycle, you can use the basic cycle for bread with extra ingredients. At the point when I need to attempt an alternate taste or shading for my bread, I add additional items like onions and nuts toward the beginning of the cycle. That way, it is totally pummeled and breaks down into the mixture when the manipulating activity is complete.

Variety

This element was normal in the more seasoned models. This cycle runs for about the very measure of time that the essential cycle runs. It has a pointer blare and furthermore shows the sign to "shape" at the subsequent ascent, so the batter can be eliminated, filled and formed the hard way, and afterward got back to the baking search for gold last ascent and baking. This cycle can likewise be utilized for a monkey bread or cinnamon twirl. If your machine does not have this feature, you can get it by programming the basic cycle, pause to interrupt the cycle after the second rise, remove the dough and shape, then return it to the baking pan and press Start to resume cycle and bake the bread.

Dough

This setting is otherwise called the Rise or Manual cycle. It is perfect for

when you want to mix and rise dough in the machine, then remove the dough, shape it by hand, and bake it in your oven. The setting with the briefest mixture cycle is Toastmaster at 1 hour and 3 minutes with 60 minutes, 30 minutes
as the normal, while the Panasonic brand is the longest cycle at 2 hours, 30 minutes (counting Preheat). Mixtures that are ready on this cycle are intended to be molded into customary portions or into unique shapes like egg turns, cloverleaf supper rolls, pizza, breadsticks, croissants, or bagels, and prepared in the stove. You can change your beloved plans for this cycle, and involving amounts that will fit in your machine. At the point when the alarm blares, eliminate the mixture and adhere to the guidelines in the menu to begin forming. In this cycle, there's occasionally an arrangement for the further choices of fundamental mixture or fast dough.

Whole Wheat

Also known as the essential wheat mode entire grain, it permits weighty entire grain flours to have a long plying time and a rising time somewhat longer than the fundamental cycle rising time, delivering a portion that is lighter and higher. It is particularly suggested for 100% entire grain or entire wheat bread, and for bread that is made of specialty flours like grain or spelt. You can likewise have the decision of essential or speedy settings inside the cycle. On a significant number of the fresher models, their pointer alarms have been inbuilt to such an extent that it blares to show when you should add any additional fixings like raisins or nuts, during the cycle. A portion of the models that have the preheat choice toward the start of their cycle generally preheat during the entire wheat cycle.

French Bread

A fresh, European, or Homemade setting is typically accessible for a similar reason. This cycle is by and large popular and generally welcomed by clients of bread machine baking. This setting is reasonable for dry nation bread with zero sugar and fat since they require a more extended time span to rise and it likewise manages the cost of the yeast a drawn-out period of time to accomplish its work. More established bread machines regularly have this cycle and it for the most part goes on for seven hours, which would be ideal for a conventional cook from France. It is additionally great for sourdough bread that contains yeast. The baking temperature of this cycle is around 325 °F. The bread prepared utilizing this cycle is generally fresh with a delicate inward crumb.

One Hour Cycle

The one hour cycle is one more kind of abbreviated cycle that produces bread inside 60 minutes. The one hour cycle takes out more than one ascent and is significantly more fast than speedy yeast bread. Like the fast yeast bread, the one hour cycle requires the utilization of moment or speedy ascent yeast. Your owner's
 manual will give data on the most proficient method to control the yeast in a formula for this cycle. I have by and by saw a reduction in taste and quality in bread made with this cycle, so I don't underwrite utilizing it. The one hour cycle can be supplanted with the speedy yeast cycle when making sans gluten yeast bread.
Bake Only

In more current models of bread machine, a heat just cycle is now and again customized so a batter ready on the mixture cycle can be molded into wanted structures and afterward got back to the machine for baking. It can likewise be utilized for a cinnamon whirl bread, a hand-blended batter, a business mixture, or if you at first intended to prepare your batter in the ordinary broiler yet altered your perspective. At the point when a cycle closes and your batter isn't as expected done, the heat just cycle is significant and you can program it to prepare in increases for as long as two hours. Assuming you are doing various sorts of baking this cycle works best.

Program

Certain machines have a capacity that permits a manual difference in the process durations to your inclination while having the option to increment manipulating rising or baking time as you want it. You can likewise program in the occasions for every one of your plans to such an extent that when you utilize a specific formula, you don't have to program the time any longer, albeit this element is just utilized by individuals who have become master cooks and are capable with the essential cycles.

Jam

Some fresher machines have an element where you can add little new natural product jams, with or without gelatin, and simultaneously make organic product margarine and chutneys. Make jam just in a machine intended for that reason to forestall spills or leakage.

Delay Feature

This is a typical and popular component since you can program the machine around evening time and have new bread in the first part of the day or meet new bread when you return home from work. There are some recipes that are not suitable for this cycle, such as recipes that include fresh ingredients like milk, cheese, eggs, fresh vegetables, and bacon, as they can become harmful at room temperature and turn sour or even result in food poisoning. The bread that requires dry milk and powdered eggs are reasonable for use with the defer clock. For ideal outcomes while utilizing the postpone clock, ensure the yeast doesn't interact with the salt (since it would control its rising power) nor interact with any fluid (it would enact it before the blending started) when the fixings are together in the bread container. Pour the liquid ingredients before any other, the salt should come after, then the dry fixings and the yeast should come toward the end. Or on the other hand change the request up to suit your machine prerequisites. Many bread machine manuals demand this precautionary measure for all plans, yet it is possibly required when utilizing the deferral timer.

Preheat

Some bread machines have a preheat or rest period setting which helps to keep ingredients put in the machine at uniform temperature by the time mixing starts just like how we used to warm flour on the oven door to encourage good rising and allow the yeast to perform at optimum capacity. This stage goes from 15 to 30 minutes and the machine will hush up during this stage since the cutting edge is latent. A portion of the more complicated machines permit you to overlook this element however others don't. It is inbuilt in each baking cycle on certain machines, while others like Breadman machines just have it on their entire wheat cycle. Certain individuals accept this component creates better bread and like this element, and some would rather avoid this is on the grounds that it builds the hour of the entire process.

Crust Control

This is a setting that provides you with the choice of light, medium, or dim covering as well as having the option to pick the cycle for your portion. It does this by somewhat changing the baking temperature or timing marginally. That way, you get to choose the completed look of your portion. The covering setting additionally impacts how all around good done a portion is on the grounds that it changes the baking time and temperature.

The Most Common Ingredients

Flour

Flour is the primary element for any bread item. The sort of flour you pick will have an effect in the portion you prepare. What's more with regards to picking flour, there are so many sorts it tends to be overpowering. But what you need to pay attention to is the amount of Protein: in the flour: the higher the flour's Protein: content, the bigger the flour's gluten-forming potential in the dough. Furthermore gluten in bread is the construction that holds the portion together and gives bread its exceptional texture.

Which flour to use?
There are five fundamental assortments of flour utilized when baking bread..

All-purpose flour contains up to 12% gluten and is ideal for use in most baked goods. Try to get unbleached options for baking bread (unbleached indicates that the flour has not been chemically treated to be whitened).

.

Whole wheat flour is more abundant in nutrients because it includes some of the grain's germ and bran. Always check the packing of the flour to ensure it is 100% whole wheat and not blended with anything else. It gives off very nutty flavors, making it ideal for nut and seed loaves or traditional whole wheat bread. This particular flour contains up to 13% gluten. Whole wheat flour creates denser loaves with more natural textures, and when baked tends to have a chewy crust.

.

Bread flour will be your go-to flour when making bread unless the recipe stipulates otherwise. It contains roughly 14% gluten and provides the baker with a more pliable dough, which in turn creates a lighter bread. Most times, all-purpose flour may be substituted with bread flour, but note that it may require more liquid because of the gluten percentage.

White whole wheat flour is a flour that is relatively new to the market. It is created using white spring wheat that is sweeter than standard wheat varieties and is lighter in color. It has a gluten percentage of 12%. It may be useful when wanting to substitute

.Yeast

all-reason flour with a better choice. It likewise has a gentle taste, which is extraordinary when you wish to add spices or different flavors to your bread. Rye flour is processed from entire rye grains, berries, or grass. Rye flour works on the dietary substance of bread portions. Customarily, rye flour is utilized to make rye or sourdough bread. Rye flours might come in three assortments: light, medium, and dim. The lighter they are, the less wheat has been left in the flour after creation. The hazier the rye flour is, the more grain has been abandoned. Hazier rye is more nutritious and delightful than lighter rye. Since rye flour doesn't have similar gluten as different flours (truth be told, it contains an alternate Protein: structure by and large), it must be blended in with universally handy or bread flour. If not, the portion will be dense.

Yeast is a key fixing that causes bread to extend and become milder and lighter. Yeast permits generally heated products to rise. Yeast rapidly retains dampness, making it transform sugar and starch into carbon dioxide. The little air pockets of gas permit the mixture to develop and increment in size.

What sort of yeast to use?
Bread machine yeast (otherwise called quick ascent yeast) and moment dry

yeast become dynamic much quicker than dynamic dry yeast and are more qualified for use in a bread machine. You can involve dynamic dry yeast in a bread machine too (truth be told, you'll see a few plans in this cookbook call for precisely dynamic dry yeast), but dynamic dry yeast isn't suggested for one-hour or express cycles, as it needs more opportunity to activate.

Additionally, I would suggest that you possibly purchase yeast when you really want it and recommend that you utilize another bundle each time you intend to prepare something. Yeast is an exceptionally sensitive item and makes for troublesome putting away on the grounds that air changes its capacity to work effectively.

Liquid (typically water, milk, or powder milk mixed in with water)

The fluid in the batter is one of the fundamental fixings answerable for enacting every one of the things inside your batter blend. It breaks up the yeast and salt, hydrates the starch and the proteins. The fluid is responsible for the consistency of the dough.
 The temperature of the fluid you use for baking bread is basic. Keep in mind, the yeast that makes the bread rise is a living life form. Assuming you use water that is excessively hot, there's a danger of killing the yeast. Assuming you utilize a fluid that is too chilly, the yeast won't enact as expected. A typical guideline is to utilize tepid water or some other liquid.

You can utilize water straightforwardly from the tap, however assuming you speculate your regular water is excessively hard, or high in chlorine, then, at that point, have a go at utilizing filtered water.

Salt
 Many individuals question the need of salt in bread baking. The short

response to that is indeed, it 's important. Bread Without salt would be boring, and it won't permit different fixings and fragrances to sing. Additionally, salt plays as an inhibitor to the yeast in the bread mixture. It eases back the rising system of the batter, which gives the gluten sufficient opportunity to fortify and create, bringing about a superior outside layer and a superior piece. Also, it adds to the kind of the bread. Without salt, an essential portion will taste dull, level, and to some degree papery.

Others:
 Oil and Butter
 Oil has various capacities with regards to baking and that incorporates

conveying the flavors, broadening the newness of the prepared products, and improving the surface. Oil likewise helps with regards to the massaging system, making the mixture more malleable and simpler to work with.

Using extra-virgin olive oil instead of standard vegetable oil is a decent decision as it conveys with it various wellbeing benefits.

Butter holds numerous properties which incorporate, adding flavor, improving the time span of usability of the item, keeping bread sodden, and advancing a more extravagant texture.

Softened margarine is ideal, as it permits the bread creator to agitate the fixings and make a smoother batter. Never use margarine directly from out of the fridge without allowing it to mellow first. A quicker method for doing as such is to put it in the microwave for an extremely brief timeframe. Or then again you can basically avoid the margarine with regards to the fridge to arrive at room temperature.

Sugar

Sugar is definitely not a fundamental fixing in bread baking. You can make fundamental regular bread with a long rising time with no sugars. Notwithstanding, aside from its improving impact on cakes and prepares, sugar plays a significant part to play in the baking process.

It can be essentially clarified. As you presumably definitely know, the course of the batter rising and growing is called maturation. It's the point at which the yeast eats the sugar in the batter and creates gases that fill the mixture with air, accomplishing delicate and feathery bread in the end.

Today, in light of the fact that the baking system has been abbreviated, in certain plans adding a smidgen of sugar can help during the maturation of the batter: sugar takes care of the yeast, bringing about a quicker rise. It doesn't need to be refined sugar. Assuming a formula requires sugar, go ahead and substitute it with a better choice, for example:

Honey Maple

.

syrup
 Molasses

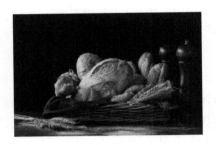

CHAPTER 2:

Classic, Traditional, and Daily Bread

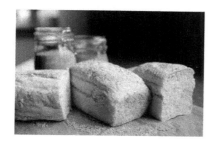

1. Mustard-Flavored General Bread

Preparation Time: 2 hours 10 minutes
Cooking Time: 40 minutes
Servings: 2 portions
Ingredients:

.

1¼ cups milk

.

3 tbsp. sunflower milk

.

3 tbsp. sour cream

.

2 tbsp. dry mustard

.

1 whole egg beaten

.

½ sachet sugar vanilla

.

4 cups flour

.

1 tsp. dry yeast

.

2 tbsp. sugar

.

2 tsp. salt

Directions:

1. Take out the bread creator's pail and pour in milk and sunflower oil; mix and afterward put the acrid cream and beaten egg.
2. Put flour, salt, sugar, mustard powder, vanilla sugar, and blend well.
3. Make a little score in the flour and sprinkle the yeast.
4. Transfer the can to your bread producer and cover.
5. Set your bread machine's program to essential/white bread and set hull type to medium.
6. Press start.
7. Wait until the cycle completes.
8. Once the portion is prepared, take the can out and allow the portion to cool for 5 minutes.
9. Gently shake the can to eliminate the loaf.
10. Transfer to a cooling rack, cut, and serve.

Nutrition:

.

Calories: 340

.

Carbohydrates: 54 g

.

Fat: 10 g

.

Protein: 10 g

2. Country White Bread

Preparation Time: 3 hours
 Cooking Time: 45 minutes
 Servings: 2 loaves
Ingredients:

.

2 tsp. active dry yeast

.

1 1/2 tbsp. sugar

.

2 cups bread flour

.

1 large egg

.

1 1/2 tsp. salt

.

1 cup warm milk, with a temperature of 110-115 °F (43 to 46 °C)

.

1 1/2 tbsp. butter

Directions:

1. Place every one of the fluid fixings in the skillet. Put every one of the dry fixings, with the exception of the yeast. Use your hand to make an opening in the focal point of the dry fixings. Put the yeast in the hole.

2. Secure the container in the chamber and cover the top. Select the fundamental setting and your favored outside shading. Press starts.
3. Once done, move the prepared bread to a wire rack. Cut once cooled.

Nutrition:
.

Calories: 105
Total Carbohydrate: 0 g Total Fat: 0 g

.

Protein: 0 g

3. Oatmeal Bread

Preparation Time: 3 hours
Cooking Time: 45 minutes
Servings: 2 portions
Ingredients:

.

3 tsp. bread machine

yeast 4 tsp. vital wheat
gluten

.

4 cups bread

.

flour 1 tsp. salt

.

1 cup instant or regular

.

oatmeal 2 tbsp. maple syrup

.

2 tbsp. unsalted butter, cubed

.

1/3 cup water, with a temperature of 80 to 90 °F(26 to 32 °C)

.

1 1/2 cups buttermilk, with a temperature of 80 to 90 °F(26 to 32 °C)

Directions:

1. Put the fixings in the dish in a specific order: buttermilk, water, spread, maple syrup, oats, salt, flour, gluten, and yeast.
2. Secure the container in the machine, cover the top, and turn it on.
3. Select the fundamental setting and your favored hull tone and press start.
4. Place the heated bread on a wire rack and permit cooling before slicing.

Nutrition:

.

Calories: 269

.

Fat: 4 g

.

Carbohydrate: 49 g

4. Anadama Bread

Preparation Time: 3 hours
Cooking Time: 45 minutes
Servings: 2 portions
Ingredients:

.

1/2 cup sunflower seeds

.

4 1/2 cups bread flour

.

3/4 cup yellow cornmeal

.

2 tsp. bread machine yeast

.

1/4 cup molasses

.

2 tbsp. unsalted butter, cubed

.

1/4 cup dry skim milk powder

.

1 1/2 cups water, with a temperature of 80 to 90 °F(26 to 32 °C)

.

1 1/2 tsp. salt

Directions:

1. Place all fixings in the skillet, with the exception of the sunflower seeds, in a specific order: water, molasses, milk, salt, margarine, cornmeal, flour, and yeast.

2. Put the dish in the machine and cover the lid.
3. Add the sunflower seeds to the leafy foods dispenser.
4. Turn the machine on and select the essential setting and your ideal shade of the outside layer. Press start.

Nutrition:

.

Calories: 130

.

Fat: 2 g

.

Carbohydrate: 25 g

.

Protein: 3 g

5. Coconut Flour Bread

Preparation Time: 10 minutes
Cooking Time: 15 minutes
Servings: 12

Ingredients: .

6 eggs

.

1/2 cup coconut flour

.

2 tbsp. psyllium husk

.

1/4 cup olive oil

.

1 1/2 tbsp. salt

.

1 tbsp. xanthan gum

.

1 tbsp. baking powder

.

2 1/4 tbsp. yeast

Directions:

1. Mix every dry fixing, with the exception of the yeast in a little blending bowl.
2. In the bread machine skillet add all the wet ingredients.
3. Add your dry fixings in general, from the little blending bowl to the bread machine dish. Top with the yeast.
4. Place the bread machine in the fundamental bread setting.
5. When the bread is done, eliminate the bread machine dish from the bread machine.
6. Once done, move the prepared bread to a wire rack. Cut once cooled.
7. The bread can be put away as long as 4 days on the counter and as long as 90 days in the freezer.

Nutrition:

.

Calories: 174

.

Fat: 15 g

.

Carbohydrates: 4 g

6. Apricot Oat

Preparation Time: 1 hour 25 minutes Cooking Time: 25 minutes
Servings: 1 portion
Ingredients:

.

4 1/4 cups bread flour

.

2/3 cup rolled oats

.

1 tbsp. white sugar

.

2 tsp. active dry

.

yeast 1 1/2 tsp. salt

.

1 tsp. ground

.

cinnamon 2 tbsp.
 butter, cut up

.

1 2/3 cups orange juice

.

1/2 cup diced dried apricots

.

2 tbsp. honey, warmed

Directions:

1. Into the dish of the bread machine, put the bread fixings in the request recommended by the maker. Then, at that point, mope in dried apricots before the work cycle completes.

2. Immediately eliminate bread from the machine when it's done and afterward coat with warmed honey. Let to cool totally before serving.

Nutrition:

.

Calories: 80

.

Fat: 2.3 g

.

Carbohydrate: 14.4 g

.

Protein: 1.3 g

---

7. Buttermilk White Bread

Preparation Time: 2 hours 50 minutes
Cooking Time: 25 minutes
Servings: 1 portion
Ingredients:

- 1 1/8 cups water

- 3 tsp. honey

- 1 tbsp. margarine

- 1 1/2 tsp. salt

- 3 cups bread flour

- 2 tsp. active dry yeast

- 4 tsp. powdered buttermilk

Directions:

1. Place all fixings as proposed by the maker into the skillet of the bread machine.

2. Choose medium hull and white bread settings. You can utilize less yeast during the sticky and blistering a very long time of summer.

Nutrition:

.

Calories: 34

.

Fat: 1 g

.

Carbohydrate: 5.7 g

.

Protein: 1 g

8. English Muffin Bread

Preparation Time: 2 hours 30 minutes
Cooking Time: 15 minutes
Servings: 2 portions
Ingredients:

.

3 cups all-purpose flour

.

2 1/4 tsp. active dry

.

yeast 1/2 tbsp. white
sugar

.

1 tsp. salt

.

1/8 tsp. baking powder

.

1 cup warm milk

.

1/4 cup water

Directions:

1. Put the fixings into the bread machine container as per the producer's suggestions. Set the machine to the batter cycle.
2. Separate the mixture into 2 inconsistent divides and afterward structure into portions. Put one part in a 9 x 5-inches portion skillet and the other in a 7 x 3-inches portion dish it's prescribed to utilize non-stick container albeit lubed and floured typical dish will be sufficient. Cover the dish and let the mixture ascend until multiplied in size.
3. Bake for around 15 minutes at 205 °C (400 °F). My grandma for the most part heats for longer to have a more sautéed and chewier crust.

Nutrition:

Calories: 64

Fat: 0.4 g

Carbohydrate: 12.8 g

Protein: 2.1 g

---

9. Homemade Wonderful Bread

Preparation Time: 3 hours 25 minutes
Cooking Time: 15 minutes
Servings: 2 portions
Ingredients:

2 1/2 tsp. active dry yeast

1 tbsp. white sugar

.

1/4 cup warm water (110 °F/45 °C)

.

4 cups all-purpose flour

.

1/4 cup dry potato

.

flakes 1/4 cup dry milk

.

powder 2 tsp. salt

.

1/4 cup white sugar

.

2 tbsp. margarine

.

1 cup warm water (110 °F/45 °C)

Directions:

1. Prepare the yeast, 1/4 cup warm water, and sugar to whisk and afterward let it sit in 15 minutes.
 2. Take all fixings along with yeast combination to place in the container of bread machine as indicated by the suggested request of assembling. Pick essential and light hull setting.

Nutrition:

.

Calories: 162

.

Fat: 1.8 g

.

Carbohydrate: 31.6 g

.

Protein: 4.5 g

10. Honey White Bread

Preparation Time: 3 hours 25 minutes
 Cooking Time: 15 minutes
 Servings: 1 portion
 Ingredients:

.

1 cup milk

.

3 tbsp. unsalted butter, melted

.

2 tbsp. honey

.

3 cups bread flour

.

3/4 tsp. salt

.

3/4 tsp. vitamin c powder

.

3/4 tsp. ground ginger

.

1 1/2 tsp. active dry yeast

Directions:

1. Follow the request as coordinated in your bread machine manual on the best way to collect the fixings. Utilize the setting for the essential bread cycle.

Nutrition:

.

Calories: 172

.

Fat: 3.9 g

.

Carbohydrate: 28.9 g

.

Protein: 5 g

11. Basic White Bread

Preparation Time: 1 hour 15 minutes
Cooking Time: 50 minutes (20+30 minutes)
Servings: 1 loaf
Ingredients:

.

½ to 5/8 cup water

.

5/8 cup milk

.

1 ½ tbsp. butter or margarine

.

3 tbsp. sugar

.

1 ½ tsp. salt

.

3 cups bread flour

.

1 ½ tsp. active dry yeast

Directions:

1. Place all fixings in the bread dish, utilizing an insignificant proportion of fluid recorded in the recipe.
2. Select medium covering setting and press start.
3. Observe the batter as it works. Following 5 to 10 minutes, when it appears to be dry and firm, or then again assuming that your machine appears like it's stressing to ply, put more fluid 1 tbsp. at a time until dough structures well.
4. Remove bread from the container once the baking cycle closes, and permit cooling before slicing.

Nutrition:

- Calories: 64

- Fat: 1 g

- Carbohydrates: 12 g

- Protein: 2 g

12. All-Purpose White Bread

Preparation Time: 2 hours 10 minutes
Cooking Time: 40 minutes
Servings: 1 portion
Ingredients:

- ¾ cup water at 80 °F

- 1 tbsp. melted butter, cooled

-

1 tbsp. sugar

.

¾ tsp. salt

.

2 tbsp. skim milk powder

.

2 cups white bread flour

.

¾ tsp. instant yeast

Directions:

1. Put all fixings into your bread machine, warily adhering to the directions of the manufacturer.
2. Set your bread machine's program to essential/white bread and set outside type to Medium.
3. Press start.
4. Wait until the cycle completes.
5. Once the portion is prepared, move the can out and allow the portion to cool for 5 minutes.
6. Gently shake the can to eliminate the loaf.
7. Place in a cooling rack, cut, and serve.

Nutrition: .

Calories: 140

.

Fat: 2 g

.

Carbohydrates: 27 g

.

Protein: 44 g

.

Fiber: 2 g

13. Crusty Sourdough Bread

Preparation Time: 15 minutes; multi week (Starter) Cooking Time: 3 hours
Servings: 1 portion
Ingredients:

.

1/2 cup water

.

3 cups bread

flour 2 tbsp.
sugar

1 ½ tsp. salt

1 tsp. bread machine or quick active dry yeast

Directions:

1. Measure 1 cup of starter and remaining bread fixings, add to bread machine pan.
2. Choose fundamental/white bread cycle with medium or light hull color.

Nutrition:

Calories: 165

Fat: 0 g

Carbohydrate: 37 g

Protein: 5 g

---

14. Multigrain Sourdough Bread

Preparation Time: 15 minutes; multi week (Starter) Cooking Time: 3 hours
Servings: 1 portion
Ingredients:

.

2 cups sourdough starter

.

2 tbsp. butter or olive

.

oil 1/2 cup milk

.

1 tsp. salt

.

1/4 cup honey

.

1/2 cup sunflower seeds

1/2 cup millet or 1/2 cup amaranth or 1/2 cup quinoa

.

3 1/2 cups multi-grain flour

Directions:

1. Add fixings to bread machine pan.
2. Choose the batter cycle.
3. Conventional Oven:
4. When a cycle is done, eliminate mixture and spot it on a delicately floured surface, and shape it into a loaf.
5. Place in a lubed portion skillet, cover, and ascend until bread is a few creeps over the edge.
6. Bake at a temperature of 375 °F or 40 to 50 minutes.

Nutrition:

.

Calories: 110

.

Fat: 1.8 g

.

Carbohydrate: 13.5 g

.

Protein: 2.7 g

---

15. Czech Sourdough Bread

Preparation Time: 15 minutes; multi week (Starter) Cooking Time: 3 hours
Servings: 1 portion
Ingredients:

.

1 cup non-dairy milk

.

1 tbsp. salt

.

1 tbsp. honey

.

1 cup sourdough starter

.

1 1/2 cups rye flour

.

1 cup bread flour

3/4 cup wheat flour

1/2 cup grated half-baked potato

5 tbsp. wheat gluten

2 tsp. caraway seeds

Directions:

1. Add fixings to bread machine pan.
2. Choose the mixture cycle.
3. The mixture should ascend, as long as 24 hours, in the bread machine until copies in size.
4. After rising heat in the bread machine for one hour.

Nutrition:

Calories: 198

Fat: 0.8 g

Carbohydrate: 39.9 g

.

Protein: 6.5 g

16. French Sourdough Bread

Preparation Time: 15 minutes; multi week (Starter) Cooking Time: 3 hours
Servings: 2 portion
Ingredients:

.

2 cups sourdough starter

.

1 tsp. salt

.

1/2 cup of water

.

4 cups white bread flour

.

2 tbsp. white cornmeal

Directions:

1. Add fixings to bread machine dish, saving cornmeal for later.
2. Choose the batter cycle.
3. Conventional Oven:
4. Preheat stove to 375 degrees.
5. At end of the batter cycle, turn the batter out onto a floured surface.
6. Add flour assuming that the batter is sticky.
7. Divide batter into 2 partitions and level into an oval shape 1 ½ inch thick.
8. Fold ovals in half longwise and squeeze creases to elongate.
9. Sprinkle cornmeal onto a baking sheet and spot the portions crease side down.
10. Cover and let ascend in until about doubled.
11. Put a shallow container of boiling water on the lower rack of the oven;
12. Use a blade to make shallow, slanting cuts in highest points of loaves
13. Put the portions in the broiler and shower with a fine water sir. Splash the broiler dividers as well.
14. Repeat showering multiple times at one-minute intervals.
15. Remove dish of water following 15 minutes of baking
16. Fully heat for 30 to 40 minutes or until brilliant brown.

Nutrition:

.

Calories: 937

.

Fat: 0.4 g

.

Carbohydrate: 196 g

Protein: 26.5 g

CHAPTER 3:

Whole Wheat and Whole Grain Bread

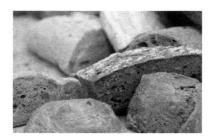

17. Whole Wheat Bread

Preparation Time: 9 minutes
 Cooking Time: 4 hours
 Servings: 12 cuts Ingredients:

.

1 cup lukewarm water

.

½ cup unsalted butter,

.

melted 2 eggs, at room

.

temperature 2 teaspoons
  table salt

.

¼ cup sugar

.

1½ cups whole-wheat flour

.

2½ cups white bread flour

.

2¼ teaspoons bread machine yeast

.

12 slice bread (1½ pounds)

.

¾ cup lukewarm water

.

⅓ cup unsalted butter, melted

.

2 eggs, at room temperature

.

1½ teaspoons table salt

.

3 tablespoons sugar

.

1 cup whole-wheat flour

.

2 cups white bread flour

.

1 ⅔ teaspoons bread machine yeast

Directions:

1. Add the water and olive oil to your machine, trailed by half of the flour.

2. Now apply the salt, sugar, dried milk powder, and remaining flour.

3. Make somewhat well or plunge at the highest point of the flour. Then, at that point, cautiously place the yeast into it, ensuring it doesn't come into contact with any liquid.

4. Set the entire feast or entire wheat setting as indicated by your machine's manual, and modify the hull setting to your particular liking.

5. Once heated, cautiously eliminate the bowl from the machine and eliminate the portion, putting it on a wire rack to cool. I don't really want to add any fixings to this specific portion, yet you can, obviously, investigation and add whatever you want.

6. Once cool, eliminate the oar; and, for the absolute best outcomes, cut with a serrated bread blade. Enjoy!

Nutrition:

.

Calories: 160

.

Fat: 31 g

.

Carbs: 30.1 g

.

Protein: 5 g

18. Toasted Almond Whole Wheat Bread

Preparation Time: 10 minutes
Cooking Time: 3 hours
Servings: 12 Ingredients:

- 1 cup, in addition to 2 tablespoons water 3

- tablespoons agave nectar

- 2 tablespoons spread, unsalted 1 1/2 cups bread

- flour

- 1 1/2 cups entire wheat flour

- 1/4 cup fragmented almonds, toasted 1 teaspoon

- salt

- 1 1/2 teaspoons speedy dynamic dry yeast

Directions:

1. Add each of the fixings in bread machine container as per the pattern in which they show up above, saving yeast.
2. Make a well in the focal point of the dry fixings and add the yeast.
3. Select the Basic cycle, light or medium covering tone, and press Start.
4. Remove heated bread from dish and cool on a rack before slicing.

Nutrition:
Calories: 150
Fat: 3.4 g
.Carbs: 26.5 g .Protein: 4.4 g

19. Whole Wheat Peanut Butter and Jelly Bread

Preparation Time: 10 minutes
Cooking Time: 3 hours
Servings: 12 cuts Ingredients:

.

1 cup water at 90 °F-100 °F (320 °C-370 °C)

.

1 ½ tablespoons vegetable oil

.

½ cup peanut butter

.

½ cup Strawberry jelly (or any preferable jelly)

.

1 tablespoon white sugar

.

1 teaspoon salt

.

1 cup whole wheat flour

.

2 cups bread flour

.

1 ½ teaspoons active dry yeast

Directions:

1. As you prep the bread machine skillet, add the accompanying in this specific request: water, jam, salt, peanut butter, earthy colored sugar, baking powder, baking pop, gluten, entire wheat flour, and yeast.

2. Choose 1 ½ Pound Loaf, Medium Crust, Wheat cycle, and afterward start the machine.
3. Once heated, place it on a rack to cool and afterward serve.
4. Enjoy!

Nutrition:

Calories: 230

.

Fat: 6 g

.

Carbs: 39 g

.

Protein: 9 g

20. Bread Machine Ezekiel Bread

Preparation Time: 10 minutes
Cooking Time: 3 hours
Servings: 12 cuts Ingredients:

.

½ cup milk

.

½ cup water

.

2 ½ tablespoons olive oil,

.

divided 1 egg

.

1 tablespoon honey

.

1 tablespoon dry lentils

.

1 tablespoon dry black beans

.

1 tablespoon dry kidney

.

beans 1 tablespoon barley

.

1 cup whole wheat flour

.

1 cup unbleached all-purpose flour

.

¼ cup millet flour

.

¼ cup cracked wheat

.

¼ cup rye flour

.

2 tablespoons wheat

.

germ 1 teaspoon salt

.

2 teaspoons bread machine yeast

Directions:

1. Soak all beans and grains in discrete dishes overnight.
2. Boil the dark beans, dry kidney beans for around 60 minutes, and afterward add lentils, millet, and grain. Then, bubble for 15 minutes more.
3. Assemble bubbled fixings in a food processor and blend until mashed.
4. Spread water into the bread machine dish, add 2 tbsp. of olive oil and honey, and afterward add the flour, raw grain. In one corner, add
salt in another yeast and start the mixture cycle.
5. When the bread machine signals, add the crush to the batter and press the entire wheat cycle. Enjoy!

Nutrition:

.

Calories: 192

.

Fat: 5 g

.

Carbs: 31 g

.

Protein: 6 g

21. Honey-Oat-Wheat Bread

Preparation Time: 10 minutes Cooking
Time: 3 hours and 45 minutes Servings:
16 slices
Ingredients:

- 1 cup buttermilk

- 1 egg

- 1/4 cup warm water (110 degrees F/45 degrees C)

- 2 tablespoons honey

- 1 1/2 cups whole wheat

- flour 1 1/2 cups all-purpose

- flour 1/2 cup quick cooking
  oats

- 2 tablespoons vegetable

oil 1 1/2 teaspoons salt

1 1/2 teaspoons active dry yeast

Directions:

1. Place the accompanying into the dish of a bread machine: yeast, sugar, and water. Allow the yeast to break up and froth for around 10 minutes. Meanwhile, consolidate the universally handy flour, powdered milk, entire wheat flour, salt, and moved oats in a bowl. Pour the margarine, honey, and vegetable oil into the yeast blend. Then add the flour mixture on top.

2. Choose the batter cycle and afterward press the beginning button. Allow the bread to machine completely finish the cycle, which traverses roughly 1 ½ hour. Put the batter into a 9x5-inches portion container that is covered with cooking splash. Pass on the bread to ascend in a warm spot for 1 hour.
3. Preheat the oven.
4. Bake for roughly 35 minutes in the warmed broiler until the top

becomes brilliant brown.
5. Enjoy!
Nutrition:

Calories: 281 Fat: 9 g

Carbs: 45 g Protein: 6 g

22. Butter Up Bread

Preparation Time: 10 minutes
Cooking Time: 3 hours
Servings: 12 cuts Ingredients:

.

3 cups bread flour

.

½ cup margarine, melted

.

1 ½ buttermilk at 110°F (450 °C)

.

½ tsp. sugar

.

1 and ¾ tsp. active dry yeast

.

1 egg at room temperature

.

1 tsp.salt

Directions:

1. Prepare the bread machine dish by adding buttermilk, softened margarine, salt, sugar, flour, and yeast in the request determined by your manufacturer.

2. Select fundamental/white setting and press start.
3. Once heated, move onto wire racks to cool before slicing.
4. Enjoy!

Nutrition:

.

Calories: 231

.

Fat: 6 g

.

Carbs: 36 g

.

Protein: 8 g

23. Butter Honey Wheat Bread

Preparation Time: 5 minutes
Cooking Time: 3 hours and 45 minutes Servings: 12 slices
Ingredients:

- 1 cup water

- 2 tablespoons margarine

- 2 tablespoons honey

- 2 cups bread flour

- 1/2 cup whole wheat

- flour 1/3 cup dry milk

- powder 1 teaspoon salt

- 1 (.25 oz.) package active dry yeast

Directions:

1. Put all ingredients into the bread machine, by way of suggested by the manufacturer.
2. For my situation, fluids generally go first.
3. Run the bread machine for a portion (1½ lbs.) overall wheat setting.
4. Once the baking system is done, move the prepared bread to a wire rack and cool before slicing.
5. Enjoy!

Nutrition:

.

Calories: 170

.

Fat: 6 g

.

Carbs: 27 g

.

Protein: 3 g

24. Molasses Wheat Bread

Preparation Time: 10 minutes or less
Cooking Time: 1 hour 30 minutes
Servings: 10
Ingredients:
8 cuts/1 pound

·

¼ cup milk, at 80 °F

·

½ cup water, at 80 °F - 90 °F 2

·

tsp. melted butter, cooled 2

·

tbsp. honey

·

1 tbsp. molasses

·

1 tsp. sugar

·

1 tbsp. skim milk powder

·

½ tsp. salt

.

1 tsp. unsweetened cocoa powder 1

.

cup white bread flour

.

1¼ cups whole-wheat flour

.

1 tsp. bread machine yeast or instant yeast

12 slices/ 1½ pounds

.

⅓ cup milk, at 80 °F

.

¾ cup water, at 80 °F - 90 °F 1

.

tbsp. melted butter, cooled 3¾

.

tbsp. honey

- 2 tbsp. molasses

- 2 tsp. sugar

- 2 tbsp. skim milk powder

- ¾ tsp. salt

- 2 tsp. unsweetened cocoa powder

- 1¾ cups whole-wheat flour

- 1¼ cups white bread flour

- 1 ⅛ tsp. bread machine yeast or instant yeast

16 slices/ 2 pounds

·

1 cup water, at 80 °F to 90 °F

·

½ cup milk, at 80 °F

·

2 tbsp. melted butter,

·

cooled 5 tbsp. honey

·

3 tbsp. molasses

·

1 tbsp. sugar

·

3 tbsp. skim milk powder

·

1 tsp. salt

.

1 tbsp. unsweetened cocoa

.

powder 2½ cups whole-wheat
 flour

.

2 cups white bread flour

.

1½ tsp. instant or bread machine yeast

Directions:

1. Place all fixings in the bread machine as recommended by the manufacturer.
 2. Set the machine for essential/white bread, select light or medium hull, and press start.
 3. When the portion is done, eliminate the can from the machine.
 4. Cool for 5 minutes.
 5. Shake the pail somewhat to eliminate the portion, and turn it out onto a rack to cool.
 6. Ingredient tip: Look for unsulphured molasses since it is better and comes up short on slight substance taste of sulphured items. Additionally, this bread is best with tacky, rich dull or blackstrap molasses rather than light-hued molasses.

Nutrition:

.

Calories: 164

.

Fat: 2 g

.

Carbohydrates: 34 g

.

Protein: 4 g

25. 100 Percent Whole-Wheat Bread

Preparation Time: 10 minutes or less
 Cooking Time: 45 minutes
 Servings: 10
 Ingredients:
 8 cuts/1 pound

.

¾ cup water, at 80 °F to 90 °F

.

1½ tbsp. melted butter, cooled

.

1½ tbsp. honey

.

¾ tsp. salt

.

2 cups whole-wheat bread flour

.

1 tsp. bread machine or instant yeast

12 slices/ 1½ pounds

.

1 ⅛ cups water, at 80 °F to 90 °F

.

2¼ tbsp. melted butter, cooled

.

2¼ tbsp. honey

.

1 ⅛ tsp. salt

.

3 cups whole-wheat bread flour

.

1½ tsp. bread machine or instant yeast

16 slices/ 2 pounds

.

1½ cups water, at 80 °F - 90 °F

.

3 tbsp. melted butter, cooled

.

3 tbsp. honey

.

1½ tsp. salt

.

3¾ cups whole-wheat bread flour

.

2 tsp. instant or bread machine yeast

Directions:

1. Place fixings in your bread machine as proposed by the manufacturer.

2. Set the machine for entire wheat/entire grain bread, select light or medium outside, and press Start.

3. When the portion is done, eliminate the container from the machine. Cool for 5 minutes.

4. Shake the can marginally to eliminate the portion, and turn it out onto a rack to cool.

" Did You Know?" Whole-wheat flour contains the whole wheat berry endosperm, grain, and microorganism - not at all like white flour, which is comprised of just the endosperm. This implies entire wheat flour is very nutritious and loaded with solid fiber, nutrients, and minerals.

Nutrition:

.

Calories: 146

.

Fat: 3 g

.

Carbohydrates: 27 g

.

Protein: 3 g

26. Cornmeal Whole Wheat Bread

Preparation Time: 1 hour and 30 minutes
 Cooking Time: 30 minutes
Servings: 10
Ingredients:

.

2 ½ tbsp. active dry yeast

.

1 1/3 cups of water

.

2 tbsp. of sugar

.

1 lightly beaten egg

.

2 tbsp. butter

.

1 ½ tbsp. of salt

.

¾ cup cornmeal

.

¾ cup whole wheat flour

.

2 ¾ cups bread flour

Directions:

1. Place all fixings into the bread machine container as indicated by the bread machine maker's instructions.
2. Select essential bread setting then, at that point, chooses medium outside and start.
3. Once the portion is done, eliminate the portion dish from the machine.
4. Allow it to cool for 10 minutes. Cut and serve.

Nutrition:

.

Calories: 228

.

Fat: 3.3 g

.

Carbs: 41.2 g

.

Protein: 7.1 g

27. Buttermilk Wheat Bread\

Preparation Time: 8 minutes
 Cooking Time: 4 hours and 30 minutes
 Servings: 16 slices
Ingredients:

.

1 1/2 cups buttermilk

.

1 1/2 tablespoons butter, melted

.

2 tablespoons white sugar

.

3/4 teaspoon salt

.

3 cups all-purpose flour

.

1/3 cup whole wheat flour

1 1/2 teaspoons active dry yeast

Directions:

1. Place all fixings in the bread machine container in the request the producer recommends.
2. Set the bread machine to the essential White Bread setting and press start.
3. After a couple of moments, put more buttermilk in the event that the fixings don't shape a ball. Assuming it's excessively free, apply a small bunch of flour.
4. One heated, let the bread cool on a wire rack before slicing.
5. Enjoy!

Nutrition:

Calories: 141

Fat: 2.5 g

Carbs: 26 g

Protein: 5 g

28. Cracked Fit and Fat Bread

Preparation Time: 5 minutes
 Cooking Time: 3 hours and 25 minutes
 Servings: 16 slices
 Ingredients:

.

1 1/4 cups water

.

2 tablespoons margarine,

.

softened 2 tablespoons dry milk
 powder

.

2 tablespoons brown

.

sugar 1 1/4 teaspoons salt

.

3 cups bread flour

1/3 cup whole wheat flour

1/4 cup cracked wheat

1 1/4 teaspoons active dry yeast

Directions:

1. In the bread machine container, measure all parts as per the producer's recommended order.
2. Choose essential/white cycle, medium outside layer, and 2 lbs. weight of portion, and afterward press start.
3. Place in a cooling rack, cut, and serve.
4. Enjoy!

Nutrition:

Calories: 65

Fat: 1 g

Carbs: 12.4 g

Protein: 2 g

29. Crunchy Honey Wheat Bread

Preparation Time: 7 minutes
 Cooking Time: 3 hours and 30 minutes
Servings: 12 slices
Ingredients:

.

1 ¼ cup warm water at 110 ₀F (450 °C)

.

2 tbsp. vegetable oil

.

3 tbsp. honey

.

1 ½ tsp. salt

.

2 cups bread flour

.

1 ½ cup whole wheat flour

.

½ cup granola

.

1(0.25 ounce) package active dry yeast

Directions:

1. Place the fixings into the bread machine following the request suggested by the manufacturer.
2. Choose the entire wheat setting or the mixture cycle on the machine. Press the beginning button.
3. Once the machine has completed the entire pattern of baking the bread in the broiler, structure the batter and add it into a portion dish that is lubed. Allow it to ascend in volume in a warm spot until it turns out to be twofold its size. Embed into the preheated 350 °F (175 °C) stove and heat for 35-45 minutes.
4. Enjoy!

Nutrition:

.

Calories: 199

.

Fat: 4.2 g

.

Carbs: 37 g

.

Protein: 6.2 g

---

30. Easy Home Base Wheat Bread

Preparation Time: 10 minutes Cooking
Time: 3 hours and 50 minutes Servings:
12 slices
Ingredients:

.

1 cup whole wheat flour

.

1 cup bread flour

.

2 tablespoons butter softened

.

1 cup warm water at 90°F (32°C)

.

1 cup warm milk at 90°F (32°C)

1 tablespoon active dry yeast

1 egg, at room temperature

1 tablespoon salt

3 tablespoons honey

Directions:

1. Add the fixings into the dish of the bread machine following the request proposed by the manufacturer.
2. Use the entire wheat cycle, pick the covering tone, weight, and start the machine.
3. Check how the mixture is working following five minutes pass since you might have to add possibly one tbsp. of water or one tbsp. of flour-in light of consistency.
4. When the bread is finished, cool it on a wire rack before slicing.
5. Enjoy!

Nutrition:

Calories: 180

Fat: 2 g

Carbs: 33 g

Protein: 7 g

31. Whole Wheat Yogurt Bread

Preparation Time: 10 minutes Cooking
 Time: 3 hours and 40 minutes Servings:
 12 slices
 Ingredients:

.

¼ tsp. ground nutmeg (optional)

.

2/3 cup water

.

¼ cup butter, melted

.

1/3 cup plain yogurt

.

2 tbsp. dry milk

.

1/3 cup honey

.

1 tbsp. active dry yeast

.

1 cup whole wheat flour

.

2 cups bread flour

.

¼ tsp. ground cinnamon

.

1 tsp. salt

Directions:

1. Start by emptying fixings into the bread dish in the guidance your maker underwrites. For my situation, fluids generally go first.

2. So, I start with water, spread, yogurt, honey, strainer flour, dry milk, add salt, ground cinnamon, and yeast in various corners of the pan.

3. Choose the entire grain setting light or medium outside layer, and press start.

4. When prepared, cool it, and afterward serve.

5. Enjoy!

Nutrition:

.

Calories: 158

.

Fat: 5 g

.

Carbs: 20 g Protein: 6 g

.

Chapter 4: Grain, Seed, and Nut Bread

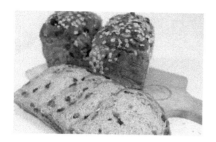

32. High Flavor Bran Bread

Preparation Time: 3 hours
Cooking Time: 15 minutes
Servings: 15
Ingredients:

.

1 1/2 cups warm water (110 °For 45 °C

.

) 2 tbsp. dry milk powder

.

2 tbsp. vegetable

.

oil 2 tbsp. molasses

.

2 tbsp. honey

.

1 1/2 tsp. salt

.

1/4 cups whole wheat flour

.

1 1/4 cups bread flour

.

1 cup whole bran cereal

.

2 tsp. active dry yeast

Directions:

1. Add the fixings in the skillet of your bread machine, as coordinated by the machine's maker.
2. Set the machine to either the entire grain or entire wheat setting.

Nutrition:

.

Calories: 146

Fat: 2.4 g

Carbohydrate: 27.9 g

Protein: 4.6 g

33. Sunflower & Flax Seed Bread

Preparation Time: 5 minutes
Cooking Time: 3 hours
Servings: 10 cuts Ingredients:

-

1 1/3 cups of water

-

2 tbsp. butter

-

3 tbsp. honey

-

1 ½ cups bread flour

.

1 1/3 cups whole wheat flour

.

1 tsp.. of salt

.

1 tsp. active dry yeast

.

½ cup flax seeds

.

½ cup sunflower seeds

Directions:

1. Add all fixings aside from sunflower seeds into the bread machine pan.
2. The select essential setting then, at that point, chooses light/medium hull and press start.
3. Add sunflower seeds not long before the last manipulating cycle.
4. Once the portion is done, eliminate the portion container from the machine. Permit it to cool for 10 minutes. Cut and serve. **Nutrition:**

Calories: 220 Fat: 5.7 g
Carbs: 36.6 g Protein: 6.6 g

34. Nutritious 9-Grain Bread

Preparation Time: 5 minutes
Cooking Time: 2 hours
Servings: 10 cuts Ingredients:

-

3/4 cup + 2 tbsp. warm water

-

1 cup whole wheat flour.

-

1 cup bread flour

-

½ cup 9-grain cereal crushed

-

1 tsp. of salt

-

1 tbsp. of butter

-

2 tbsp. of sugar

.

1 tbsp. milk powder

.

2 tsp. active dry yeast

Directions:

1. Put all fixings into the bread machine.
2. The select entire wheat setting then, at that point, chooses light/medium outside and start.
3. Once the portion is done, eliminate the portion dish from the machine.
4. Permit it to cool for 10 minutes. Cut and serve.

Nutrition:

.

Calories: 132

.

Fat: 1.7 g

.

Carbs: 25 g

.

Protein: 4.1 g

35. Oatmeal Sunflower Bread

Preparation Time: 15 minutes Cooking Time: 3 hours 30 minutes Servings: 10 slices
Ingredients:

- 1 cup of water

- ¼ cup of honey

- 2 tbsp. butter

- softened 3 cups bread flour

- ½ cup old fashioned oats

- 2 tbsp. milk powder

1 ¼ tsp. of salt

2 ¼ tsp. active dry yeast

½ cup sunflower seeds

Directions:

1. Add all fixings aside from sunflower seeds into the bread machine pan.
2. The select fundamental setting then, at that point, chooses light/medium outside layer and press start. Add sunflower seeds not long before the last manipulating cycle.
3. Once the portion is done, eliminate the portion container from the machine. Permit it to cool for 10 minutes. Cut and serve.

Nutrition:

Calories: 215

Fat: 4.2 g

Carbs: 39.3 g

Protein: 5.4 g

---

36. Delicious Cranberry Bread

Preparation Time: 5 minutes
 Cooking Time: 3 hours 27 minutes
 Servings: 10 slices
Ingredients:

.

1 ½ cup warm

.

water 2 tbsp. brown

.

sugar 1 ½ tsp. of salt.

.

2 tbsp. olive

.

oil 4 cups flour

.

1 ½ tsp. cinnamon

.

1 ½ tsp. cardamom

.

1 cup dried

.

cranberries 2 tsp. yeast

Directions:

1. Put all fixings into the bread machine in the recorded order.
2. Select sweet bread setting then, at that point, select light/medium outside layer and start. When the portion is done, eliminate the portion skillet from the machine.
3. Allow it to cool for 20 minutes. Cut and serve.

Nutrition:

.

Calories: 223

.

Fat: 3.3 g

.

Carbs: 41.9 g

.

Protein: 5.5 g

---

37. Coffee Raisin Bread

Preparation Time: 15 minutes
Cooking Time: 3 hours
Servings: 10 cuts Ingredients:

.

2 ½ tsp. active dry yeast

.

¼ tsp. ground cloves

.

¼ tsp. ground allspice

.

1 tsp. ground cinnamon

.

3 tbsp. of sugar

.

1 lightly beaten egg

.

3 tbsp. olive oil

.

1 cup strong brewed coffee

.

3 cups bread flour

.

3/4 cup raisins

.

1 ½ tsp. of salt

Directions:

1. Add all fixings aside from raisins into the bread machine pan.
2. The select essential setting then, at that point, chooses light/medium outside layer and press start. Add raisins not long before the last plying cycle.
3. Once the portion is done, eliminate the portion container from the machine. Permit it to cool for 10 minutes. Cut and serve.

Nutrition:

Calories: 230

Fat: 5.1 g

Carbs: 41.5 g

Protein: 5.2 g

---

38. Healthy Multigrain Bread

Preparation Time: 5 minutes
Cooking Time: 40 minutes
Servings: 10 cuts Ingredients:

1 ¼ cups of water

2 tbsp. of butter

1 1/3 cups bread flour

.

1 ½ cups whole wheat flour

.

1 cup multigrain cereal

.

3 tbsp. brown sugar

.

1 ¼ tsp. of salt

.

2 ½ tsp. yeast

Directions:
1. Put fixings recorded in the bread machine container. Select essential bread setting then, at that point, select light/medium covering and start.
2. Once the portion is done, eliminate the portion dish from the machine. Permit it to cool for 10 minutes. Cut and serve. **Nutrition:**

.

Calories: 159

.

Fat: 2.9 g

.

Carbs: 29.3 g

.

Protein: 4.6 g

39. Italian Pine Nut Bread

Preparation Time: 5 minutes
Cooking Time: 3 hours 30 minutes
Servings: 10 slices
Ingredients:

.

1 cup + 2 tbsp. of water

.

3 cups bread flour

.

2 tbsp. of sugar

.

1 tsp. of salt

1 1/4 tsp. active dry yeast

1/3 cup basil pesto

2 tbsp. flour

1/3 cup pine nuts

Directions:
1. In a little compartment, join basil pesto and flour and blend until very much mixed. Add pine nuts and mix well. Add water, bread flour, sugar, salt, and yeast into the bread machine pan.

2. The select fundamental setting then, at that point, chooses medium hull and press start. Add basil pesto blend not long before the last working cycle.

3. Once the portion is done, eliminate the portion container from the machine. Permit it to cool for 10 minutes. Cut and serve. **Nutrition:**

Calories: 180

Fat: 3.5 g

Carbs: 32.4 g

Protein: 4.8 g

40. Whole Wheat Raisin Bread

Preparation Time: 5 minutes
 Cooking Time: 2 hours
 Servings: 10 cuts Ingredients:

.

3 ½ cups whole wheat flour

.

2 tsp. dry yeast

.

2 lightly beaten eggs

.

¼ cup butter softened

.

3/4 cup of water

.

1/3 cup of milk

.

1 tsp. of salt

.

1/3 cup of sugar

.

4 tsp. cinnamon

.

1 cup raisins

Directions:

1. Add water, milk, margarine, and eggs to the bread skillet. Add remaining fixings aside from yeast to the bread pan.
2. Make a little opening into the flour with your finger and add yeast to the opening. Ensure yeast won't be blended in with any liquids.
3. The select entire wheat setting then, at that point, chooses light/medium outside and start. When the portion is done, eliminate the portion skillet from the machine.
4. Allow it to cool for 10 minutes. Cut and serve.

Nutrition:

Calories: 290

Fat: 6.2 g

Carbs: 53.1 g

Protein: 6.8 g

41. Healthy Spelt Bread

Preparation Time: 15 minutes Cooking Time: 40 minutes Servings: 10 cuts Ingredients:

1 ¼ cups of milk.

2 tbsp. of sugar

2 tbsp. olive oil

.

1 tsp. of salt.

.

4 cups spelled flour

.

2 ½ tsp. yeast

Directions:

1. Add all fixings as per the bread machine maker's guidelines into the bread machine.
2. Select essential bread setting then, at that point, select light/medium outside and start. When the portion is done, eliminate the portion container from the machine.
3. Allow it to cool for 10 minutes. Cut and serve.

Nutrition:

.

Calories: 223

.

Fat: 4.5 g

.

Carbs: 40.3 g

.

Protein: 9.2 g

---

42. Honey and Flaxseed Bread

Preparation Time: 3 hours
Cooking Time: 15 minutes
Servings: 12
Ingredients:

.

1 1/8 cups water

.

1 1/2 tbsp. flaxseed oil

.

3 tbsp. honey

.

1/2 tbsp. liquid lecithin

.

3 cups whole wheat flour

- 1/2 cup flax seed

- 2 tbsp. bread flour

- 3 tbsp. whey

- powder 1 1/2 tsp. sea salt

- 2 tsp. active dry yeast

Directions:

1. In the bread machine skillet, put in each of the fixings following the request suggested by the manufacturer.
2. Choose the wheat cycle on the machine and press the beginning button to run the machine.

Nutrition:

- Calories: 174

Fat: 4.9 g

.

Carbohydrate: 30.8 g

.

Protein: 7.1 g

---

43. Honey Wheat Bread

Preparation Time: 3 hours 5 minutes
Cooking Time: 15 minutes
Servings: 10
Ingredients:

.

1 1/8 cups warm water (110 °F /45 °C)

.

3 tbsp. honey

.

1/3 tsp. salt

.

1 1/2 cups whole wheat

.

flour 1 1/2 cups bread flour

.

2 tbsp. vegetable oil

.

1 1/2 tsp. active dry yeast

Directions:

1. Put the fixings into the bread machine following the request suggested by the manufacturer.
2. Choose the wheat bread cycle and the setting for light tone on the machine.

Nutrition: .

Calories: 180

.

Fat: 3.5 g

.

Carbohydrate: 33.4 g

Protein: 5.2 g

44. Maple Whole Wheat Bread

Preparation Time: 3 hours 5 minutes
Cooking Time: 15 minutes
Servings: 10
Ingredients:

.

1/2 cups whole wheat flour

.

1/2 cup bread flour

.

1/3 tsp. salt

.

1 1/4 cups water

.

4 tbsp. maple syrup

.

1 tbsp. olive oil

.

1 1/2 tsp. active dry yeast

Directions:

1. Put the fixings into the bread machine dish following the request recommended by the manufacturer.
2. Choose the wheat bread cycle on the machine and press the beginning button.

Nutrition:

.

Calories: 144

.

Fat: 2.8 g

.

Carbohydrate: 26.9 g

.

Protein: 4.3 g

45. Super Seed Bread

Preparation Time: 5 minutes
Cooking Time: 22 min
Serving: 7
Ingredients:

.

2/3 cup entire psyllium husk

.

1/4 cup chia seeds

.

1/4 cup pumpkin seeds

.

1/4 cup hemp or sunflower seeds

.

3 sp. ground sesame seeds or ground flaxseeds

.

1 tsp. preparing powder

.

1/4 tsp. salt

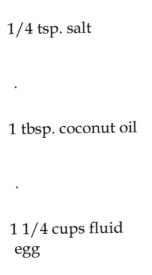

1 tbsp. coconut oil

1 1/4 cups fluid
egg

1/2 cup unsweetened almond milk

Directions:

1. In an enormous mixing bowl, incorporate each and every dry fixing and mix well. You can make your own ground sesame seeds by blending them until they're a fine powder.

2. Melt the coconut oil in the microwave (around 30 seconds), add it to the dry mix and blend well. By then incorporate 1/4 cup liquid egg whites and 1/2 cup unsweetened almond milk. Mix well and let the mix address 10-15 minutes while you preheat your oven to 325° F.

3. Wet some material paper under warm water and shake it off, by then press it into a 9" x 5" bread tin. Incorporate your mix and press it into the edges of the tin. You can in like manner add a few extra seeds to the most elevated place of the mix here. Trim the overflow material paper and put it on the oven for 70 minutes.

4. Slice the entire part and let cool on a drying rack. This bread can discharge on the off chance that not cut at the earliest open door and left to cool on a
rack.

Nutrition:

Cal: 70

Fat: 8 g

Carbs: 4 g

Protein: 8 g

---

46. Chia Seed Bread

Preparation Time: 10 minutes
Cooking Time: 3 hours 30 minutes
Servings: 14 slices
Ingredients:

¼ cup chia seeds

¾ cup hot water

- 2 ⅜ cups water

- ¼ cup oil

- ½ lemon, zest, and juice

- 1¾ cups white flour

- 1¾ cups whole wheat flour

- 2 tbsp. baking powder

- 1 tbsp. salt

- 1 tbsp. sugar

2½ tbsp. quick-rise yeast

Directions:

1. Add the chia seeds to a bowl, cover with boiling water, blend well and let them remain until they are drenched and coagulated, and don't feel warm to touch.

2. Add every fixing to the bread machine in the request and at the temperature suggested by your bread machine manufacturer.
3. Close the top, select the essential bread, medium outside setting on your bread machine, and press start.
4. When the blending sharp edge quits moving open the machine and blend everything by hand with a spatula.
5. When the bread machine has completed the process of baking eliminate the bread and put it on a cooling rack.

Nutrition:

Calories: 152

Fat: 2 g

Carbs: 28 g

Protein: 6 g

47. Corn, Poppy Seeds and Sour Cream Bread

Preparation Time: 2 hours 40 minutes
 Cooking Time: 50 minutes
 Servings: 2 portions
 Ingredients:

.

3½ cups wheat flour

.

1¾ cups corn flour

.

5 ounces sour cream

.

2 tablespoons corn oil

.

2 teaspoons active dried yeast

.

2 teaspoons salt

16 ¼ ounces water

·

¼ cup poppy seeds for sprinkling

Directions:

1. Add 16¼ ounces of water and corn oil to the bread producer bucket.
2. Add flour, acrid cream, sugar, and salt from various angles.
3. Make a furrow in the flour and add yeast.
4. Set the program of your bread machine to Basic/White Bread and set hull type to Medium.
5. Press START.
6. Wait until the cycle completes.
7. Once the portion is prepared, take the can out and allow the portion to cool for 5 minutes.
8. Gently shake the pail to eliminate the loaf.
9. Moisten the surface with water and sprinkle with poppy seeds. 10. Transfer to a cooling rack, cut, and serve.

Nutrition:
Calories: 374 Cal
Fat: 10 g
Carbohydrates: 64 g
Protein: 9 g

CHAPTER 5:

Herb and Spice Bread

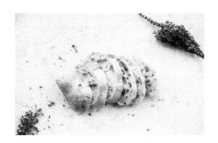

48. Italian Herb Bread

Preparation Time: 5 minutes Cooking
Time: 3 hours and 5 minutes Servings:
14 slices
Ingredients:

·

2 tbsp. margarine

·

2 tbsp. sugar

·

1½ cups
water

·

3 tbsp. powdered milk

.

1½ tbsp. dried

.

marjoram 1½ tbsp. dried basil

.

1½ tbsp. salt

.

4 cups bread

.

flour 1¼ tbsp.
 yeast

.

1½ tbsp. dried thyme

Directions:

1. Place every fixing to the bread machine in the guidance and at the temperature suggested by your bread machine manufacturer.

2. Close the top, pick the fundamental bread, medium outside layer setting on your bread machine, then, at that point, press start.

3. If the bread machine has completed the process of baking eliminate the bread.

4. Put it on a cooling rack.

Nutrition:

.

Calories:120

.

Fat: 3 g

.

Carbs: 20 g

.

Protein: 4 g

49. Caramelized Onion Bread

Preparation Time: 15 minutes Cooking
Time: 3 hours and 35 minutes Servings:
14 slices
Ingredients:

.

½ tbsp. butter

.

½ cup onions sliced

.

1 cup of water

.

1 tbsp. olive oil

.

3 cups Gold Medal Better

.

1 tbsp. salt

.

1¼ tbsp. quick active dry yeast

Directions:

1. Melt the spread through medium-low hotness in a skillet.
2. Cook the onions in the margarine for 10 to 15 minutes until they are brown and caramelized - then, at that point, eliminate from the heat.
3. Add every fixing with the exception of the onions to the bread machine.
4. Choose the essential bread, medium outside setting on your bread machine, and press start.
5. Add ½ cup of onions 5 to 10 minutes before the last plying cycle ends.
6. When the bread machine has finished baking eliminate the bread and put it on a cooling rack.

Nutrition:

Calories:160 Fat: 3 g Carbs: 30 g
Protein: 4 g

50. Olive Bread

Preparation Time: 10 minutes
Cooking Time: 3 hours
Servings: 14 cuts Ingredients:

.

½ cup brine from the olive jar

.

Add warm water (110 °F) to make 1½ cup when combined with brine

.

2 tbsp. olive oil

.

3 cups bread flour

.

1 2/3 cups whole wheat

.

flour 1 ½ tbsp. salt

.

2 tbsp. sugar

.

1 1/2 tbsp. dried leaf

.

basil 2 tbsp. active dry
yeast

.

2/3 cup finely chopped Kalamata olives

Directions:

1. Add every fixing with the exception of the olives to the bread machine.

2. Close the top, select the wheat, medium outside layer setting on your bread machine, and press start.

3. Add the olives 10 minutes before the last massaging cycle ends.

4. When the bread machine has gotten done with baking get the bread and put it on a cooling rack.

Nutrition:

·

Calories:140

·

Fat: 1 g

·

Carbs: 28 g

·

Protein: 5 g

51. Dilly Onion Bread

Preparation Time: 10 minutes Cooking Time: 3 hours and 5 minutes Servings: 14 slices

Ingredients:

·

¾ cup water (70 °F to 80 °F)

.

1 tbsp. butter softened

.

2 tbsp. sugar

.

3 tbsp. dried minced onion

.

2 tbsp. dried parsley flakes

.

1 tbsp. dill weed

.

1 tbsp. salt

.

1 garlic clove, minced

.

2 cups bread flour

.

1/3 cup whole wheat flour

.

1 tbsp. nonfat: dry milk powder

.

2 tbsp. active dry yeast serving

Directions:

1. Add every fixing to the framework in the request and at the temperature suggested by your bread machine manufacturer.
2. Cover the top, select the essential bread, medium outside set on your bread machine, and press start.
3. When the bread machine has total baking eliminate the bread and put it on a cooling rack.

Nutrition:

.

Calories:77

.

Fat: 1 g

.

Carbs: 16 g

.

Protein: 3 g

52. Original Italian Herb Bread

Preparation Time: 15 minutes
Cooking Time: 3 hours

.

Servings: 20 cuts Ingredients:

.

1 cup water at 80 °F

.

½ cup olive brine

.

1½ tbsp. butter

.

3 tbsp. sugar

2 tsp. salt

.

5 1/3 cups flour

.

2 tsp. bread machine yeast

.

20 olives, black/green

.

1½ tsp. Italian herbs

Directions:

1. Cut olives into slices.
2. Put all fixings into your bread machine (aside from olives), cautiously adhering to the guidelines of the manufacturer.
3. Put the program of your bread machine to French bread and set covering type to medium.
4. Once the creator blares, add olives.
5. Wait until the cycle completes.
6. Once the portion is done, take the can out and cool the portion for 6 minutes.
7. Wobble the can to take off the loaf.

Nutrition:

.

Calories: 386 Fat: 7 g

.

Carbs: 71 g

.

Protein: 10 g

---

53. Lovely Aromatic Lavender Bread

Preparation Time: 5 minutes
Cooking Time: 2 hours and 45 minutes
Servings: 8 slices
Ingredients:

.

¾ cup milk at 80 °F

.

1 tbsp. melted butter, cooled

.

1 tbsp. sugar

.

¾ tsp. salt

- 1 tsp. fresh lavender flower, chopped

- ¼ tsp. lemon zest

- ¼ tsp. fresh thyme, chopped

- 2 cups white bread flour

- ¾ tsp. instant yeast

Directions:

1. Place all fixings into your bread machine, adhering to the directions of the manufacturer.
2. Put the program of your bread machine to fundamental/white bread and set outside layer type to medium.
3. Wait until the cycle completes.
4. Once the portion is done, take the container out and allow the portion to cool for 5 minutes.
5. Shake the can marginally to eliminate the loaf.

Nutrition:

Calories: 144 Fat: 2 g

Carbs: 27 g Protein: 4 g

---

54. Cinnamon & Dried Fruits Bread

Preparation Time: 5 minutes
Cooking Time: 3 hours
Servings: 16 cuts Ingredients:

- 2¾ cups flour

- 1½ cups of dried fruits

- 4 tbsp. sugar

- 2½ tbsp. butter

- 1 tbsp. milk powder

-

1 tsp. cinnamon

.

½ tsp. ground nutmeg

.

¼ tsp. vanillin

.

½ cup peanuts

.

½ cup powdered sugar, for sprinkling

.

1 tsp. salt

.

1½ bread machine yeast

Directions:

1. Place all fixings into your bread machine (aside from peanuts and powdered sugar), cautiously adhering to the directions of the manufacturer.

2. Put the program of your bread machine to fundamental/white bread and set outside layer type to medium.

3. Once the bread creator signals, saturate mixture with a bit of water and add peanuts.

4. Wait until the cycle completes.

5. Once the portion is done, take the can out and allow the portion to cool for 5 minutes.

6. Shake the can somewhat to eliminate the loaf.

7. Sprinkle with powdered sugar.

Nutrition: .

Calories: 315

.

Fat: 4 g

.

Carbs: 65 g

.

Protein: 5 g

55. Herbal Garlic Cream Cheese Delight

Preparation Time: 5 minutes
Cooking Time: 2 hours and 45 minutes
Servings: 8 slices
Ingredients:

.

1/3 cup water at 80 °F

.

1/3 cup herb and garlic cream cheese mix, at room temp

.

1 whole egg beaten, at room temp

.

4 tsp. melted butter, cooled

.

1 tbsp. sugar

.

2/3 tsp. salt

.

2 cups white bread flour

.

1 tsp. instant yeast

Directions:

1. Add every one of the fixings to your bread machine, cautiously adhering to the directions of the manufacturer.

2. Put the program of your bread machine to fundamental/white bread and set covering type to medium.

3. Wait until the cycle completes.

4. Once the portion is done, take the can out and allow the portion to cool for 5 minutes.

5. Shake the can somewhat to eliminate the loaf.

Nutrition:

.

Calories: 182

.

Fat: 6 g

.

Carbs: 27 g

.

Protein: 5 g

56. Oregano Mozza-Cheese Bread

Preparation Time: 15 minutes Cooking
Time: 3 hours and 15 minutes Servings:
16 slices
Ingredients:

.

1 cup (milk + egg) mixture

.

½ cup mozzarella cheese

.

2¼ cups flour

.

¾ cup whole grain flour

.

2 tbsp. sugar

.

1 tsp. salt

.

2 tsp. oregano

.

1½ tsp. dry yeast

Directions:

1. Place all fixings into your bread machine, cautiously adhering to the directions of the manufacturer.
2. Put the program of your bread machine to essential/white bread and set outside type to dark.
3. Wait until the cycle completes.
4. Once the portion is done, take the can out and allow the portion to cool for 5 minutes.
5. Shake the can marginally to eliminate the loaf.
Nutrition:

Calories: 209 Fat: 2.1 g
Carbs: 40 g Protein: 7.7 g

57. Cumin Tossed Fancy Bread

Preparation Time: 5 minutes
Cooking Time: 3 hours and 15 minutes
Servings: 16 slices
Ingredients:

·

5 1/3 cups wheat flour

·

1½ tsp. salt

·

1½ tbsp. sugar

·

1 tbsp. dry

yeast 1¾ cups
 water

·

2 tbsp. cumin

·

3 tbsp. sunflower oil

Directions:

1. Add warm water to the bread machine bucket.
2. Add salt, sugar, and sunflower oil.
3. Sift in wheat flour and add yeast.
4. Put the program of your bread machine to French bread and set hull type to medium.
5. Once the producer blares, add cumin.
6. Wait until the cycle completes.
7. Once the portion is done, take the can out and allow the portion to cool for 5 minutes.
8. Shake the can somewhat to eliminate the loaf.

Nutrition:

·

Calories: 368

·

Fat: 7 g

Carbs: 67 g

·

Protein: 9.5 g

---

58. Potato Rosemary Loaf

Preparation Time: 5 minutes
Cooking Time: 3 hours and 25 minutes
Servings: 20 slices
Ingredients:

·

4 cups wheat flour

·

1 tbsp. sugar

·

1 tbsp. sunflower oil

·

1½ tsp. salt

·

1½ cups water

.

1 tsp. dry yeast

.

1 cup mashed potatoes, ground through a sieve

.

Crushed rosemary to taste

Directions:

1. Add flour, salt, and sugar to the bread producer can and join blending paddle.
2. Add sunflower oil and water.
3. Put in yeast as directed.
4. Put the program of your bread machine to bread with filling mode and set hull type to medium.
5. Once the bread producer blares and motions toward add more fixings, open the top, add pureed potatoes, and slashed rosemary.
6. Wait until the cycle completes.
7. Once the portion is done, take the can out and allow the portion to cool for 5 minutes.
8. Shake the can somewhat to eliminate the loaf.

Nutrition:
Calories: 276

.

Fat: 3 g

Carbs: 54 g

Protein: 8 g

---

59. Cardamom Cranberry Bread

Preparation Time: 5 minutes Cooking Time: 3 hours
Servings: 14 cuts Ingredients:

.

1¾ cups water

.

2 tbsp. brown

.

sugar 1½ tbsp. salt

.

2 tbsp. coconut oil

.

4 cups flour

.

2 tbsp. cinnamon

.

2 tbsp. cardamom

.

1 cup dried cranberries

.

2 tbsp. yeast

Directions:

1. Add every fixing with the exception of the dried cranberries to the bread machine in the request and at the temperature proposed by your bread machine manufacturer.

2. Close the top; select the fundamental bread setting on your bread machine and press start.
3. Add the dried cranberries 5 to 10 minutes before the last plying cycle ends.
4. When the bread machine has quit baking eliminate the bread and put it on a cooling rack.

Nutrition:

.

Calories:157

Fat: 3 g

Carbs: 41 g

Protein: 3 g

---

60. Garlic Bread

Preparation Time: 2 hours 30 minutes
Cooking Time: 40 minutes
Servings: 1 portion
Ingredients:

.

1 3/8 cups water

.

3 tbsp. olive oil

.

1 tsp. minced

.

garlic 4 cups bread

.

flour 3 tbsp. white

.

sugar 2 tsp. salt

.

1/4 cup grated Parmesan cheese

.

1 tsp. dried basil

.

1 tsp. garlic powder

.

3 tbsp. chopped fresh chives

.

1 tsp. coarsely ground black

.

pepper 2 1/2 tsp. bread machine yeast

Directions:

1. Add the fixings to the bread machine in the request recommended by your bread machine manufacturer.
2. Select the fundamental or the white bread cycle on the machine and press the beginning button.

Nutrition:

.

Calories: 175

.

Fat: 3.7 g

.

Carbohydrate: 29.7 g

.

Protein: 5.2 g

61. Cracked Black Pepper Bread

Preparation Time: 3 hours 30 minutes
Cooking Time: 15 minutes
Servings: 8
Ingredients:

- ¾ cup water, at 80 °F - 90

- °F 1 tbsp. melted butter,

- cooled 1 tbsp. sugar

- ¾ tsp. salt

- 2 tbsp. skim milk

- powder 1 tbsp. minced
  chives

- ½ tsp. garlic powder

- ½ tsp. cracked black pepper

2 cups white bread flour

¾ tsp. bread machine or instant yeast

Directions:

1. Place the fixings in the bread machine as recommended by the manufacturer.
2. Set the machine for essential/white bread, select light or medium outside, and press start.
3. Once the portion is done, take the can out and allow the portion to cool for 5 minutes.
4. Shake the can somewhat to eliminate the loaf.
5. Wrap the bread with a kitchen towel and put it away for 60 minutes. If not, you can cool it on a wire rack.

Nutrition:

Calories: 141

Fat: 2 g

Carbohydrate: 27 g

Protein: 4 g

---

62. Spicy Cajun Bread

Preparation Time: 2 hours
 Cooking Time: 15 minutes
 Servings: 8
 Ingredients:

·

¾ cup water, at 80 °F - 90

·

°F 1 tbsp. melted butter,

·

cooled 2 tsp. tomato paste

·

1 tbsp. sugar

·

1 tsp. salt

·

2 tbsp. skim milk powder

- ½ tbsp. Cajun seasoning

- ⅛ tsp. onion powder

- 2 cups white bread flour

1 tsp. bread machine or instant yeast

Directions:

1. Put all fixings in the bread machine as proposed by the manufacturer.
2. Set the machine for fundamental/white bread, select light or medium outside, and press start.
3. Once the portion is done, take the pail out and allow the portion to cool for 5 minutes.
4. Shake the container somewhat to eliminate the loaf.

Nutrition:

- Calories: 141

- Fat: 2 g

Carbohydrate: 27 g

Protein: 4 g

63. Anise Lemon Bread

Preparation Time: 2 hours
Cooking Time: 15 minutes
Servings: 8
Ingredients:

⅔ cup of water, at 80 °F to 90 °F

1 egg at room temperature

2 ⅔ tbsp. butter, melted and cooled

2 ⅔ tbsp. honey

⅓ tsp. salt

.

⅔ tsp. anise seed

.

⅔ tsp. lemon zest

.

2 cups white bread flour

.

1 ⅓ tsp. bread machine or instant yeast

Directions:

1. Put the fixings in your bread machine as recommended by the manufacturer.
2. Program the machine for essential/white bread, pick light or medium hull, and press start.
3. Once the portion is done, take the can out and allow the portion to cool for 5 minutes.
4. Shake the can marginally to eliminate the loaf.

Nutrition:

.

Calories: 158

.

Fat: 5 g

.

Carbohydrate: 27 g

.

Protein: 4 g

64. Cardamon Bread

Preparation Time: 2 hours
 Cooking Time: 15 minutes
 Servings: 8
 Ingredients:

.

½ cup of milk, at 80 °F to 90 °F

.

1 egg at room temperature

.

1 tsp. melted butter, cooled

.

4 tsp. honey

⅔ tsp. salt

⅔ tsp. ground cardamom

2 cups white bread flour

¾ tsp. bread machine or instant yeast **Directions:**

1. Place the fixings in your bread machine as recommended by the manufacturer.
2. Set the machine for essential/white bread, pick light or medium covering, and press start.
3. Once the portion is done, take the can out and allow the portion to cool for 5 minutes.
4. Shake the can marginally to eliminate the loaf.

Nutrition:

Calories: 149

Fat: 2 g

Carbohydrate: 29 g

.

Protein: 5 g

65. Rosemary Bread

Preparation Time: 5 minutes
 Cooking Time: 3 hours
 Servings: 14 cuts Ingredients:

.

1 1/3 cups milk

.

4 tbsp. butter

.

3 cups bread flour

.

1 cup one-minute oatmeal

.

1 tbsp. salt

6 tbsp. white granulated sugar

1 tbsp. onion powder

1 tbsp. dried rosemary

1 1/2 tbsp. bread machine yeast

Directions:

1. Add the fixings in the bread machine in the request and at the temperature proposed by your bread machine manufacturer.
2. Close the cover, select the fundamental bread, medium hull setting on your bread machine, and press start.
3. After the bread machine has completed the process of massaging sprinkle some rosemary on top of the bread dough.
4. Remove the bread, then, at that point, put it on a cooling rack.

Nutrition:

Calories:123

Fat: 3 g

.

Carbs: 27 g

.

Protein: 5 g

66. Chive Bread

Preparation Time: 10 minutes
Cooking Time: 3 hours
Servings: 14 cuts Ingredients:

.

2/3 cup milk (70 °F to 80 °F)

.

1/4 cup water (70 °F to 80 °F)

.

1/4 cup sour cream

.

2 tbsp. butter

- 1 1/2 tbsp. sugar

- 1 1/2 tbsp. salt

- 3 cups bread flour

- 1/8 tbsp. baking soda

- 1/4 cup minced chives

- 2 1/4 tbsp. active dry yeast leaves

Directions:

1. Add every fixing to the machine in the request and at the temperature supported by your bread machine manufacturer.
2. Close the top, pick the fundamental bread, medium outside layer setting on your bread machine, and press start.
3. When the bread machine has been done heating up eliminate the bread and put it on a cooling rack.

Nutrition:

Calories:105

Fat: 2 g

Carbs: 18 g

Protein: 4 g

67. Pumpkin Cinnamon Bread

Preparation Time: 10 minutes
Cooking Time: 3 hours
Servings: 14 cuts Ingredients:

1 cup of sugar

1 cup canned

pumpkin 1/3 cup

.

vegetable oil 1 tbsp.
vanilla

.

2 eggs

.

1 1/2 cups all-purpose bread flour

.

2 tbsp. baking powder

.

1/4 tbsp. salt

.

1 tbsp. ground

.

cinnamon 1/4 tbsp.

.

ground nutmeg 1/8 tbsp. ground cloves

Directions:

1. Place every fixing to the bread machine in the request and at the temperature embraced by your bread machine manufacturer.
2. Close the top, select the fast, medium hull setting on your bread machine, and press start.
3. When the bread machine has completed the process of baking get out the bread and put it on a cooling rack.

Nutrition:

.

Calories:140

.

Fat: 5 g

.

Carbs: 39 g

.

Protein: 3 g

68. Olive and Garlic Sourdough Bread

Preparation Time: 15 minutes; multi week (Starter) Cooking Time: 3 hours
Servings: 1 portion
Ingredients:

- 2 cups sourdough starter 3

- cups flour

- 2 tbsp. olive oil 2

- tbsp. sugar

- 2 tsp. salt

- 1/2 cup chopped black olives 6

- cloves chopped garlic

Directions:
1. Add starter and bread fixings to the bread machine pan. 2. Choose the batter cycle.
Conventional Oven:

3. Preheat broiler to 350 0F.
4. When a cycle is finished, assuming the mixture is tacky add more flour.
5. Shape batter onto a baking sheet or put into portion pan
6. Bake for 35-45 minutes until golden.
7. Cool before slicing.

Nutrition:

.

Calories: 150

.

Fat: 0.5 g

.

Carbohydrate: 26.5 g

.

Protein: 3.4 g

CHAPTER 6:

Gluten-Free

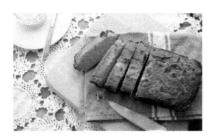

69. Gluten-Free Brown Bread

Preparation Time: 5 minutes
Cooking Time: 3 hours
Servings: 12
Ingredients:

-

2 large eggs, lightly beaten

-

1 3/4 cups warm water

-

3 tbsp. canola oil

-

1 cup brown rice flour

.

3/4 cup oat flour

.

1/4 cup tapioca starch

.

1 1/4 cups potato starch

.

1 1/2 tsp. salt

.

2 tbsp. brown sugar

.

2 tbsp. gluten-free flaxseed meal

.

1/2 cup nonfat: dry milk powder

.

2 1/2 tsp. xanthan gum

.

3 tbsp. psyllium, whole husks

.

2 1/2 tsp. gluten-free yeast for bread machines

Directions:

1. Add the eggs, water, and canola oil to the bread producer dish and mix until combined.
2. Whisk each of the dry fixings aside from the yeast together in an enormous blending bowl.
3. Add the dry fixings on highest of the wet ingredients.
4. Create a well in the center of the dry fixings and add the yeast.
5. Set Gluten-Free cycle, medium covering tone, and afterward press Start.
6. When the bread is done, lay the skillet on its side to cool prior to cutting to serve.

Nutrition:

.

Calories: 201

.

Fat: 5.7 g

.

Carbs: 35.5 g

.

Protein: 5.1 g

70. Easy Gluten-Free, Dairy-Free Bread

Preparation Time: 15 minutes Cooking
Time: 2 hours and 10 minutes Servings:
12
Ingredients:

.

1 1/2 cups warm

.

water 2 tsp. active dry

.

yeast 2 tsp. sugar

.

2 eggs, room temperature

.

1 egg white, room

temperature 1 1/2 tbsp. apple

.

cider vinegar 4 1/2 tbsp. olive
oil

.

3 1/3 cups multi-purpose gluten-free flour

Directions:

1. Start with adding the yeast and sugar to the water, then, at that point, mix to blend in a huge blending bowl; put away until frothy, around 8 to 10 minutes.

2. Whisk the two eggs and one egg white together in a different blending bowl and add to the bread creator's heating up pan.
3. Pour apple juice vinegar and oil into the baking pan.
4. Add frothy yeast/water combination to baking pan.
5. Add the multi-reason sans gluten flour on top.
6. Set for Gluten-Free bread setting and Start.
7. Remove and alter the container onto a cooling rack to eliminate the bread from the baking dish. Permit cooling totally prior to cutting to serve.
Nutrition:

Calories: 241 Fat: 6.8 g
Carbs: 41 g Protein: 4.5 g

71. Gluten-Free Sourdough Bread

Preparation Time: 5 minutes
Cooking Time: 3 hours
Servings: 12
Ingredients:

.

1 cup of water

.

3 eggs

.

3/4 cup ricotta cheese

.

1/4 cup honey

.

1/4 cup vegetable oil

.

1 tsp. cider vinegar

.

3/4 cup gluten-free sourdough starter

.

2 cups white rice flour

.

2/3 cup potato starch

.

1/3 cup tapioca flour

.

1/2 cup dry milk powder

.

3 1/2 tsp. xanthan gum

.

1 1/2 tsp. salt

Directions:

1. Combine wet fixings and fill bread producer pan.
2. Mix dry fixings in a huge blending bowl, and extra top of the wet ingredients.
3. Select the without gluten cycle and press start.
4. Remove the dish from the machine and permit the bread to stay in the prospect 10 minutes.
5. Transfer to a cooling rack before slicing.

Nutrition:
.Calories: 299 .

Fat: 7.3 g

.

Carbs: 46 g

.

Protein: 5.2 g

72. Gluten-Free Crusty Boule Bread

Preparation Time: 15 minutes
Cooking Time: 3 hours
Servings: 12
Ingredients:

.

3 1/4 cups gluten-free flour mix

.

1 tbsp. active dry yeast

.

1 1/2 tsp. kosher salt

.

1 tbsp. guar gum

.

1 1/3 cups warm water

.

2 large eggs, room temperature

.

2 tbsp., plus two tsp. olive oil

.

1 tbsp. honey

Directions:

1. Combine the dry fixings as a whole, do exclude the yeast, in a huge blending bowl; set aside.
2. Mix the water, eggs, oil, and honey in a different blending bowl.
3. Pour the wet fixings into the bread maker.
4. I am including the dry fixings top of the wet ingredients.
5. Form a well in the middle piece of the dry fixings and add the yeast.
6. Set to without gluten setting and press start.
7. Remove heated bread and permit it to cool totally. Dig out and load up with soup or plunge to use as a boule or cut for serving.

Nutrition:

.

Calories: 480

.

Fat: 3.2 g

.

Carbs: 103.9 g

.

Protein: 2.4 g

73. Simple Keto Bread

Preparation Time: 3 minutes Cooking Time: 15 minutes Servings: 8
Ingredients:

.

3 cups almond flour

.

2 tbsp. inulin

.

1 tbsp. whole milk

.

½ tbsp. salt

.

2 tbsp. active yeast

.

1 ¼ cups warm water

.

1 tbsp. olive oil

Directions:

1. Use a little blending bowl to consolidate every single dry fixing, aside from the yeast.
2. In the bread machine container add all wet ingredients.
3. Add your dry fixings in general, from the little blending bowl to the bread machine dish. Top with the yeast.
4. Set the bread machine to the fundamental bread setting.
5. When the bread is done, eliminate the bread machine skillet from the bread machine.
6. Cool somewhat then exchange it to a cooling rack.
7. The bread can be saved as long as 5 days on the counter and for as long as 90 days in the freezer.

Nutrition:

Calories: 85

Fats 7 g

Carbohydrates 4 g

Protein: 3 g

74. Classic Keto Bread

Preparation Time: 3 minutes
Cooking Time: 15 minutes
Servings: 10
Ingredients:

.

7 eggs

.

½ cup ghee

.

2 cups almond flour

.

1 tbsp. baking powder

.

¼ tbsp. salt

Directions:

1. Pour eggs and ghee into the bread machine pan.
2. Add remaining ingredients.
3. Set the bread machine to the speedy setting.
4. Allow the bread machine to finish its cycle.
5. When the bread is done, eliminate the bread machine container from the bread machine.
6. Cool somewhat then exchange it to a cooling rack.
7. The bread can be hidden away as long as 4 days on the counter and for as long as 90 days in the freezer.

Nutrition:

.

Calories: 167

.

Fats 16 g

.

Carbohydrates 2 g

.

Protein: 5 g

---

75. Collagen Keto Bread

Preparation Time: 5 minutes
 Cooking Time: 15 minutes
 Servings: 12
 Ingredients:

.

½ cup collagen protein, unflavored grass-fed

.

6 tbsp. almond flour

.

5 eggs

1 tbsp. coconut oil, melted

1 tbsp. baking powder

1 tbsp. xanthan gum

¼ tbsp. Himalayan pink salt

Directions:

1. Pour all wet fixings into the bread machine bread pan.
2. Add dry fixings to the bread machine pan.
3. Set bread machine to the sans gluten setting
4. When the bread is done, eliminate the bread machine dish from the bread machine.
5. Cool somewhat then exchange it to a cooling rack.
6. The bread can be amassed as long as 4 days on the counter and for as long as 90 days in the freezer.

Nutrition:

Calories: 77

Fats 14 g

.

Carbohydrates 6 g

.

Protein: 5 g

76. Gluten-Free Cranberry Bread

Preparation Time: 4 minutes
Cooking Time: 19 min
Servings: 8
Ingredients:

.

2 cups almond flour

.

1/2 cup powdered erythritol or

.

swerve, 1/2 tsp. Steviva stevia powder

.

see note 1 1/2 tsp. preparing powder

- 1/2 tsp. preparing pop

- 1 tsp. salt

- 4 tbsp. unsalted spread dissolved (or coconut oil)

- 1 tsp. blackstrap molasses discretionary (for dark-colored sugar season)

- 4 large eggs at room temperature

- 1/2 cup coconut milk

- 1 sack cranberries 12 ounces

Directions:

1. Preheat oven to 350 degrees; oil a 9-by-5 inches segment dish and put in a safe spot.
2. In a gigantic bowl, whisk together flour, erythritol, stevia, warming powder, planning pop, and salt; put in a safe spot.
3. In a medium bowl, merge margarine, molasses, eggs, and coconut milk.
4. Mix dry mix into wet mix until all-around joined.
5. Fold in cranberries. Void hitter into the organized skillet.
6. Bake until a toothpick implanted in the point of convergence of the part admits all, around 1 hour and 15 minutes.
7. Transfer skillet to a wire rack; let the bread cool 15 minutes prior to ousting from the dish.

Nutrition:

.

Cal: 90

.

Fat: 8 g

.

Carbs: 4 g

.

Protein: 8 g

77. Gluten-Free Chocolate Zucchini Bread

Preparation Time: 5 minutes
Cooking Time: 15 minutes
Servings: 12
Ingredients:

- 1 ½ cups coconut flour

- ¼ cup unsweetened cocoa powder

- ½ cup erythritol

- ½ tbsp. cinnamon

- 1 tbsp. baking soda

- 1 tbsp. baking powder

- ¼ tbsp. salt

- ¼ cup coconut oil, melted

4 eggs

·

1 tbsp. vanilla

·

2 cups zucchini, shredded

Directions:

1. Shred the zucchini and use paper towels to deplete overabundance water, set aside.

·

2. Lightly beat eggs with coconut oil then, at that point, add to bread machine pan.
3. Add the excess fixings to the pan.
4. Set bread machine to gluten-free.
5. When the bread is done, eliminate the bread machine container from the bread machine.
6. Cool somewhat then exchange it to a cooling rack.
7. You can store your bread for up to 5 days.

Nutrition:

·

Calories: 185 Fats 17 g

·

Carbohydrates 6 g

.

Protein: 5 g

---

78. Gluten-Free Loaf

Preparation Time: 5 minutes
Cooking Time: 15 minutes
Servings: 12
Ingredients:

.

½ cup butter, melted

.

3 tbsp. coconut oil,

.

melted 6 eggs

.

2/3 cup sesame seed flour

.

1/3 cup coconut flour

2 tbsp. baking powder

.

1 tbsp. psyllium husks

.

½ tbsp. xanthan gum

.

½ tbsp. salt

Directions:

1. Pour in eggs, softened spread, and dissolved coconut oil into your bread machine pan.
2. Add the leftover fixings to the bread machine pan.
3. Set bread machine to gluten-free.
4. When the bread is done, eliminate the bread machine dish from the bread machine.
5. Cool somewhat then exchange it to a cooling rack.
6. You can store your bread for up to 3 days.

Nutrition:

.

Calories: 146

.

Fats 14 g

Carbohydrates 1.2 g

Protein: 3.5 g

---

79. Gluten-Free Potato Bread

Preparation Time: 5 minutes
Cooking Time: 3 hours
Servings: 12
Ingredients:

·

1 medium russet potato, baked, or mashed leftovers

·

2 packets gluten-free quick yeast

·

3 tbsp. honey

·

3/4 cup warm almond milk

·

2 eggs, one egg white

.

3 2/3 cups almond flour

.

3/4 cup tapioca flour

.

1 tsp. sea salt

.

1 tsp. dried chive

.

1 tbsp. apple cider vinegar

.

1/4 cup olive oil

Directions:

1. Combine the whole dry fixings, aside from the yeast, in an enormous blending bowl; set aside.
2. Whisk together the milk, eggs, oil, apple juice, and honey in a different blending bowl.
3. Pour the wet fixings into the bread maker.
4. Add the dry fixings on top of the wet ingredients.
5. Produce a well in the dry fixings and add the yeast.
6. Set to sans gluten bread setting light covering tone, and press start.
7. Allow cooling totally before slicing.

Nutrition: .

Calories: 232

.

Fat: 13.2 g

.

Carbs: 17.4 g

.

Protein: 10.4 g

80. Sorghum Bread

Preparation Time: 5 minutes
Cooking Time: 3 hours
Servings: 12
Ingredients:

.

1 1/2 cups sorghum flour

.

1/2 cup tapioca starch

.

1/2 cup brown rice flour

.

1 tsp. xanthan gum

.

1 tsp. guar gum

.

1/3 tsp. salt

.

3 tbsp. sugar

.

2 1/4 tsp. instant yeast

.

3 eggs (room temperature, lightly beaten)

.

1/4 cup oil

.

1 1/2 tsp. vinegar

.

3/4-1 cup milk (105-115°F)

Directions:

1. Blend the dry fixings in a bowl, excluding the yeast.
2. Add the wet fixings to the bread producer container, then, at that point, add the dry fixings on top.
3. Next is making a well in the focal point of the dry fixings and add the yeast.
4. Set to fundamental bread cycle, light hull tone, and press start.
5. Remove and lay on its side to cool on a wire rack before serving.

Nutrition:

.

Calories: 169

.

Fat: 6.3 g

.

Carbs: 25.8 g

.

Protein: 3.3 g

81. Paleo Bread

Preparation Time: 10 minutes Cooking
Time: 3 hours and 15 minutes Servings:
16
Ingredients:

.

4 tbsp. chia seeds

.

1 tbsp. flax meal

.

3/4 cup, plus one tbsp. water

.

1/4 cup coconut oil

.

3 eggs, room temperature

- 1/2 cup almond milk

- 1 tbsp. honey

- 2 cups almond flour

- 1 1/4 cups tapioca flour

- 1/3 cup coconut flour

- 1 tsp. salt

- 1/4 cup flax meal

- 2 tsp. cream of

tartar 1 tsp. baking
soda

2 tsp. active dry yeast

Directions:

1. Combine the chia seeds in addition to a tbsp. of flax dinner in a blending bowl; mix in the water, and set aside.
2. Dissolve the coconut oil in a dish, and let it cool down to lukewarm.
3. Whisk in the eggs, almond milk, and honey.
4. Whisk in the chia seeds and flax supper gel and empty it into the bread producer pan.
5. Stir the almond flour, custard flour, coconut flour, salt, and 1/4 cup of flax meal.
6. Whisk the cream of tartar and baking soft drink in a different bowl and consolidate it with the other dry ingredients.
7. Put the dry fixings into the bread machine.
8. Make somewhat well on top and add the yeast.
9. Start the machine on the wheat cycle, light or medium hull tone, and press start.
10. Remove to cool totally prior to cutting to serve.

Nutrition:

Calories: 190

Fat: 10.3 g

Carbs: 20.4 g

.

Protein: 4.5 g

---

82. Gluten-Free Oat and Honey Bread

Preparation Time: 5 minutes
Cooking Time: 3 hours
Servings: 12
Ingredients:

.

1 1/4 cups warm

.

water 3 tbsp. honey

.

2 eggs

.

3 tbsp. butter, melted

.

1 1/4 cups gluten-free oats

- 1 1/4 cups brown rice

- flour 1/2 cup potato starch

- 2 tsp. xanthan

- gum 1 1/2 tsp.

- sugar 3/4 tsp. salt

- 1 1/2 tbsp. active dry yeast

Directions:

1. Add fixings in the request recorded above, with the exception of the yeast.
2. Then structure a well in the focal point of the dry fixings and add the yeast.
3. Select the without gluten cycle, light outside shading, and press start.
4. Remove bread and permit the bread to cool on its side on a cooling rack for 20 minutes prior to cutting to serve.

Nutrition:

Calories: 151

Fat: 4.5 g

Carbs: 27.2 g

Protein: 3.5 g

---

83. Gluten-Free Cinnamon Raisin Bread

Preparation Time: 5 minutes
Cooking Time: 3 hours
Servings: 12
Ingredients:

3/4 cup almond milk

2 tbsp. flax meal

- 6 tbsp. warm water

- 1 1/2 tsp. apple cider vinegar

- 2 tbsp. butter

- 1 1/2 tbsp. honey

- 1 2/3 cups brown rice flour

- 1/4 cup corn starch

- 2 tbsp. potato starch

- 1 1/2 tsp. xanthan gum

1 tbsp. cinnamon

.

1/2 tsp. salt

.

1 tsp. active dry yeast

.

1/2 cup raisins

Directions:

1. Mix flax and water and let the combination represent 5 minutes.
2. Combine dry fixings in a different bowl, aside from the yeast.
3. Add wet fixings to the bread machine.
4. Add the dry combination on top and make a well in the center of the dry mix.

5.
.Add the yeast to the well.

6. Set to sans gluten, light outside shading, and press start.
7. After the first manipulating and rise cycle, add raisins.
8. Remove to a cooling rack when heated and let cool for 15 minutes before slicing.

Nutrition:
Calories: 192

.

Fat: 4.7 g

.

Carbs: 38.2 g

.

Protein: 2.7 g

CHAPTER 7:

Cheese Bread

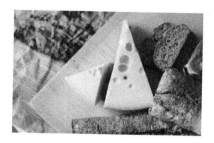

84. Cream Cheese Bread

Preparation Time: an hour
Cooking Time: 35 minutes
Servings: 1 loaf
Ingredients:

.

1/2 cup water

.

1/2 cup cream cheese, softened

.

¼ cup melted butter

.

1 beaten egg

.

3 tbsp. sugar

.

1 tsp. salt

.

3 cups bread flour

.

1 1/2 tsp. active dry yeast

Directions:

1. Place all fixings in the container in the request as suggested by your bread machine manufacturer.
2. An interaction on the mixture cycle.
3. Remove from machine, structure into a portion, and spot in lubed 9x5 portion pan.
4. Cover and let ascend until doubled.
5. Bake in a 350 F° broiler for roughly 35 minutes.

Nutrition:

.

Calories: 150

.

Fat: 5 g

.

Carbohydrate: 24 g

.

Protein: 3 g

85. Mozzarella Cheese and Salami Loaf

Preparation Time: 2 hours 50 minutes
Cooking Time: 45 minutes
Servings: 1 portion
Ingredients:

.

¾ cup water, at 80 °F

.

1/3 cup mozzarella cheese, shredded

.

2 tsp. sugar

.

2/3 tsp. salt

2/3 tsp. dried basil

·

Pinch of garlic powder

·

3 cups + 2 tbsp. white bread flour

·

1 tsp. instant yeast

·

½ cup hot salami, finely diced

Directions:

1. Add the recorded fixings to your bread machine (aside from salami), following the makes instructions.
2. Set the bread machine's program to fundamental/white bread and the outside kind to light. Press start.
3. Let the bread machine work and delay until it blares, this your sign to add the leftover fixings. Now add the salami.
4. Wait until the excess heat cycle completes.
5. Once the portion is done, take the container out and allow the portion to cool for 5 minutes.
6. Shake the pail marginally to eliminate the loaf.
7. Serve and enjoy!

Nutrition:

Calories: 164

.

Fat: 3 g

.

Carbohydrate: 28 g

.

Protein: 6 g

86. Olive and Cheddar Loaf

Preparation Time: 2 hours 50 minutes
Cooking Time: 45 minutes
Servings: 1 portion
Ingredients:

.

1 cup water, room temperature

.

1 ½ tsp. sugar

¾ tsp. salt

1 and 1/ cups sharp cheddar cheese, shredded

3 cups bread flour

1 tsp. active dry yeast

¾ cup pimiento olives, drained and sliced

Directions:

1. Add the recorded fixings to your bread machine (aside from salami), following the fabricates instructions.
2. Set the bread machine's program to essential/white bread and the hull type to light. Press start.
3. Let the bread machine work and delay until it signals, this your sign to add the excess fixings. Now add the salami.
4. Wait until the leftover heat cycle completes.
5. Once the portion is done, take the can out and allow the portion to cool for 5 minutes.
6. Shake the can somewhat to eliminate the portion. Slice.
7. Serve and enjoy!

Nutrition:

Calories: 124

.

Fat: 4 g

.

Carbohydrate: 19 g

.

Protein: 5 g

87. Three-Cheese Bread

Preparation Time: 10 minutes
 Cooking Time: 25 minutes
 Servings: 8
 Ingredients:

.

3 cups bread or all-purpose flour

.

1 1/4 cup warm milk

- 2 tbsp. oil

- 2 tbsp. sugar

- 1 tbsp. instant yeast or one packet

- 1 cup cheddar cheese

- 1/2 cup parmesan cheese

- 1/2 cup mozzarella cheese

1. Preparing the Ingredients. Place all fixings in the bread dish with the fluid dry-yeast layering.
2. Put the container in the Zojirushi bread machine.
3. Select the prepare cycle. Pick standard fundamental setting. 4. Press start and delay until the portion is cooked.
5. The machine will begin the keep warm mode after the bread is complete.
6. Let it stay in that mode for roughly 10 minutes before unplugging. 7. Remove the skillet and hang tight for it to chill off for around 10 minutes.

Nutrition:

-

Calories: 174

.

Fat: 3.1 g

.

Carbs: 31.1 g

.

Protein: 5.1 g

88. Spinach and Feta whole Wheat Bread

Preparation Time: 10 minutes
Cooking Time: 25 minutes
Servings: 8
Ingredients:

.

3 2/3 cups whole wheat flour

.

1 1/2 tbsp. instant yeast

.

1/4 cup unsalted butter, melted

.

1 cup lukewarm water

.

2 tbsp.

.

sugar 1/2
 tbsp. salt

.

3/4 cups blanched and chopped spinach, fresh

.

1/2 tbsp. pepper

.

1/2 tbsp. paprika

.

1/3 cup feta cheese, mashed

Directions:

1. Place all fixings, with the exception of spinach, spread, and feta, in the bread dish in the fluid dry-yeast layering.
2. Put the container in the Zojirushi bread machine.
3. Select the Bake cycle. Pick Regular entire wheat. Press start.
4. When the mixture has accumulated, physically add the feta and spinach.
5. Resume and delay until the portion is cooked. Once cooked, brush with butter.
6. The machine will begin the keep warm mode after the bread is complete.
7. Make it stay in that mode for around 10 minutes before unplugging.
8. Remove the container and simply cool it down for around 10 minutes.

Nutrition:

.

Calories: 174

.

Fat: 3.1 g

.

Carbs: 31.1 g

.

Protein: 5.1 g

89. Cheese Swirl Loaf

Preparation Time: 15 minutes
Cooking Time: 25 minutes
Servings: 8
Ingredients:

- 3 cups all-purpose flour

- 1 1/4 cup lukewarm milk

- 3 tbsp. sugar

- 1 tbsp. salt

- 1 1/2 tbsp. instant yeast

- 3 tbsp. melted butter

- 4 slices of Monterey cheese

- 1/2 cup mozzarella cheese

1/2 cup Edam or any quick melting cheese

1/2 tbsp. paprika

1. Place all fixings, aside from cheeses, in the bread dish in the fluid dry-yeast layering.
2. Put the skillet in the Zojirushi bread machine.
3. Select the Bake cycle. Pick Regular essential Setting. Press start. 4. Place all the cheese in a microwavable bowl. Melt in the microwave for 30 seconds. Cool, yet make a point to keep soft. 5. After 10 minutes into the manipulating system, stop the machine. Take out portion of the batter. Roll it level on the work surface. 6. Spread the cheddar on the level batter, then, at that point, roll it meagerly. Get back to the bread container carefully. 7. Resume and delay until the portion is cooked.
8. The machine will begin the keep warm mode after the bread is complete.
9. Let it stay in that mode for around 10 minutes before unplugging. 10. To end by eliminating the skillet and let it cool down for around 10 minutes.

Nutrition:

Calories: 174

Fat: 3.1 g

Carbs: 31.1 g

Protein: 5.1 g

---

90. Chili Cheese Bacon Bread

Preparation Time: 10 minutes
 Cooking Time: 25 minutes
 Servings: 8
Ingredients:

.

½ cup milk

.

1½ tsp. melted butter, cooled

.

1½ tbsp. honey

.

1½ tsp. salt

.

½ cup chopped and drained green chiles

.

½ cup (2 ounces) grated Cheddar cheese

- ½ cup chopped cooked bacon

- 3 cups white bread flour

- 2 tsp. bread machine or instant yeast

Directions:

1. Place the fixings in your Zojirushi bread machine.
2. Select the heat cycle. Program the machine for ordinary fundamental, select light or medium outside layer, and press start.
3. Remove the can from the machine.
4. Let the portion cool for 5 minutes.
5. Gently swing the can to eliminate the portion and put it out onto a rack to cool.

Nutrition:

Calories: 174 Fat: 3.1 g
Carbs: 31.1 g Protein: 5.1 g

91. Cottage Cheese Bread

Preparation Time: 2 hours 50 minutes Cooking Time: 45 minutes
Servings: 1 portion
Ingredients:

1/2 cup water

.

1 cup cottage cheese

.

1 ½ tbsp. margarine

.

1 egg

.

1 tbsp. white sugar

.

1/4 tsp. baking soda

.

1 tsp. salt

.

3 cups bread flour

.

1/2 tsp. active dry yeast

Directions:

1. Place the fixings into the bread machine, as per the request suggested by the producer, and afterward push the beginning button.

2. In the event that the mixture looks excessively tacky, go ahead and utilize around a large portion of a cup more bread flour. **Nutrition:**

.

Calories: 171

.

Fat: 3.6 g

.

Carbohydrate: 26.8 g

.

Protein: 7.3 g

92. Green Cheese Bread

Preparation Time: 3 hours

.

Cooking Time: 15 minutes
 Servings: 8
 Ingredients:

·

¾ cup lukewarm water

·

1 tbsp. sugar

·

1 tsp. kosher salt

·

½ cup green cheese

·

1 cup wheat bread machine flour

·

9/10 cup whole-grain flour, finely ground

·

1 tsp. bread machine yeast

1 tsp. ground paprika

Directions:

1. Place every one of the dry and fluid fixings, with the exception of paprika, in the container and adhere to the directions for your bread machine.

2. Pay specific regard for estimating the fixings. Utilize an estimating cup, estimating spoon, and kitchen scales to do so.
3. Dissolve yeast in warm milk in a pan and include the last turn.
4. Put the paprika after the blare or spot it in the container of the bread machine.
5. Set the baking project to fundamental and the covering type to dark.
6. If the batter is excessively thick or excessively wet, change how much flour and fluid in the recipe.
7. When the program has gotten done, remove the dish from the bread machine and let it cool for 5 minutes.
8. Shake the portion out of the skillet. If vital, utilize a spatula.
9. Wrap the bread with a kitchen towel and put it away for 60 minutes. Any other way, you can cool it on a wire rack.

Nutrition:
Calories: 118

Fat: 1 g

Carbohydrate: 23.6 g

Protein: 4.1 g

93. Cheesy Chipotle Bread

Preparation Time: 2 hours
 Cooking Time: 15 minutes
 Servings: 8
Ingredients:

.

⅔ cup water, at 80 °F to 90 °F

.

1½ tbsp. sugar

.

¾ tsp. salt

.

1½ tbsp. powdered skim milk

.

½ tsp. chipotle chili powder

.

3 cups white bread flour

½ cup (2 ounces) shredded sharp Cheddar cheese

¾ tsp. bread machine or instant yeast

Directions:

1. Place the fixings in your bread machine as suggested by the manufacturer.
2. Program the machine for essential/white bread, select light or medium covering, and press start.
3. When the portion is done, eliminate the pail from the machine.
4. Let the portion cool for 5 minutes.
5. Gently shake the container to eliminate the portion, and turn it out onto a rack to cool.

Nutrition:

Calories: 139

Fat: 1 g

Carbohydrate: 27 g

Protein: 6 g

94. Cheddar Cheese Basil Bread

Preparation Time: 2 hours
 Cooking Time: 15 minutes
 Servings: 8

 Ingredients: .

⅔ cup milk, at 80 °F to 90 °F

.

1 tbsp. melted butter, cooled

.

1 tbsp. sugar

.

⅔ tsp. dried basil

.

½ cup (2 ounces) shredded sharp Cheddar cheese

.

½ tsp. salt

.

3 cups white bread flour

.

1 tsp. bread machine or active dry yeast

Directions:

1. Place the fixings in your bread machine as suggested by the manufacturer.
2. Program the machine for fundamental/white bread, select light or medium outside layer, and press start.
3. When the portion is done, eliminate the can from the machine.
4. Let the portion cool for 5 minutes.
5. Gently shake the can to eliminate the portion, and turn it out onto a rack to cool.

Nutrition:

.

Calories: 166

.

Fat: 4 g

.

Carbohydrate: 26 g

.

Protein: 6 g

95. Olive Cheese Bread

Preparation Time: 2 hours
 Cooking Time: 15 minutes
Servings: 8
Ingredients:

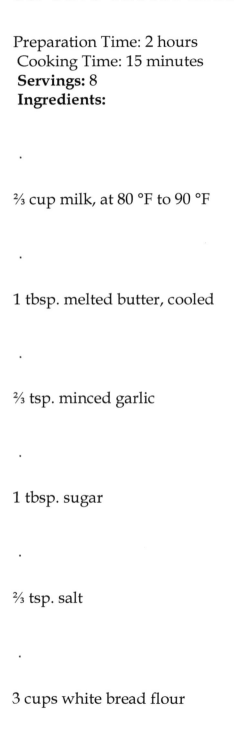

.

⅔ cup milk, at 80 °F to 90 °F

.

1 tbsp. melted butter, cooled

.

⅔ tsp. minced garlic

.

1 tbsp. sugar

.

⅔ tsp. salt

.

3 cups white bread flour

.

½ cup (2 ounces) shredded Swiss cheese

.

¾ tsp. bread machine or instant yeast

.

¼ cup chopped black olives

Directions:

1. Place the fixings in your bread machine as suggested by the manufacturer.
2. Program the machine for fundamental/white bread, select light or medium hull, and press start.
3. When the portion is done, eliminate the can from the machine.
4. Let the portion cool for 5 minutes.
5. Gently shake the can to eliminate the portion, and turn it out onto a rack to cool.

Nutrition:

.

Calories: 175

.

Fat: 5 g

.

Carbohydrate: 27 g

.

Protein: 6 g

CHAPTER 8:

Pizza and Focaccia Dough

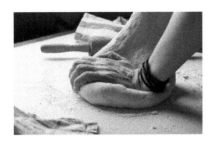

96. Easiest Focaccia Recipe

Preparation Time: 30 minutes
Cooking Time: 50 minutes
Servings: 4
Ingredients:

.

1 tsp. white sugar

.

1 (.25 oz.) package active dry yeast

.

1/3 cup warm water (110 °F /45 °C

) 2 cups all-purpose flour

.

2 tbsp. olive

.

oil 1/4 tsp. salt

Directions:

1. Dilute sugar and yeast in warm water in a little bowl. Put away for 10 minutes until the combination becomes creamy.
 2. Mix completely the yeast blend and flour until all around joined. Step by step add water 1 tbsp. at a time until all flour is ingested. At the point when the mixture becomes unblemished, dust with flour the work surface and momentarily manipulate the batter for around 1 minute.
 3. Put the mixture in a daintily oiled enormous bowl and give the mixture to cover the opposite side with oil. Utilizing a sodden material, cover the bowl and let it remain at room temperature for around 30 minutes until the volume of mixture becomes doubled.
 4. Set broiler to 475 °F (245 °C) for preheating.
 5. Punch down the batter and move it to a surface softly floured. Straighten the mixture into a sheet and move it to a baking sheet with light oil. Spread the highest point of the mixture with oil and put on some salt.
 6. In the preheated broiler, heat the focaccia for 10 to 20 minutes or until wanted freshness is accomplished, for soggy and feathery focaccia, heat for just 10 minutes, and for crispier and more obscure focaccia, prepare for 20 minutes.
 Nutrition:

Calories: 296
 Fat: 7.4 g
 Carbohydrate: 49.4 g Protein: 7.1 g

97. Stromboli Pizza

Preparation Time: 1 hour
 Cooking Time: 30 minutes
 Servings: 8
 Ingredients:

- 15 oz. all-purpose flour

- 10 oz. water

- 2 tbsp. extra-virgin olive oil

- ½ tbsp. dry yeast

- A pinch of salt

For the Stuffing:

- 10 oz. tomato sauce

.

10 oz. mozzarella cheese

.

½ cup black olives

.

12-14 salami slices

.

1 tbsp. pickled capers

.

1 tbsp. oregano

.

1 tbsp. extra virgin olive oil

.

1/8 tsp. fresh basil

.

A pinch of salt

Directions:

1. Mix the flour with yeast, water, and additional virgin olive oil until you get a smooth and versatile pizza
 2. dough
 3. Set the batter to the side until it copies in volume.
 4. Meanwhile, blend the pureed tomatoes with some olive oil, salt, and oregano to taste.
 5. Cut the olives into cuts up the mozzarella.
 6. When the batter has risen, spread it utilizing a rolling pin.
 7. Spread pureed tomatoes on top, and afterward add the tricks, olives, mozzarella, and salami. Add a fresh
 8. Basil leaves as well.
 9. Roll the mixture into a round and hollow shape and spot it in a stove plate covered with baking paper.
 10. Grease the moved pizza with additional virgin olive oil everywhere, then, at that point, heat at 350 °F for around 1 hour.
 11. When it's done, serve it cut into slices.

Nutrition:

.

Calories: 750

.

Fat: 6.1 g

.

Carbohydrate: 32 g

.

Protein: 9.6 g

CHAPTER 9:

Fast, No Yeast bread

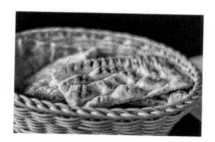

98. Keto Easy Bread

Preparation Time: 15 minutes
Cooking Time: 45 minutes
Servings: 10
Ingredients:

.

¼ tbsp. cream of tartar

.

1 ½ tbsp. baking powder (double acting)

.

4 large eggs

.

1 ½ cups vanilla whey Protein:

.

¼ cup olive oil

.

¼ cup coconut milk, unsweetened

.

½ tbsp. salt

.

¼ cup unsalted butter softened

.

12 oz. cream cheese softened

.

½ tbsp. Xanthan gum

.

½ tbsp. baking soda

Directions

1. Preheat broiler to 325 0F.
2. Layer aluminum foil over the portion container and splash with olive oil.
3. Beat the margarine with cream cheddar in a bowl until blended well.
4. Add oil and coconut milk and mix until blended. Add eggs, individually until completely blended. Set aside.
5. In a bowl, whisk whey protein, ½ tbsp. Thickener, baking pop, cream of tartar, salt, and baking powder.
6. Add combination to egg/cheddar blend and gradually blend until completely consolidated. Don't over blend.
7. Place in the broiler and prepare for 40 to 45 minutes, or until brilliant brown.
8. Cool, cut, and serve.

Nutrition:

.

Calories: 294.2

.

Fat: 24 g

.

Carb: 1.8 g

.

Protein: 17 g

99. Puri Bread

Preparation Time: 10 minutes
Cooking Time: 5 minutes
Servings: 6
Ingredients:

.

1 cup almond flour, sifted

.

½ cup of warm water

.

2 tbsp. clarified butter

.

1 cup olive oil for

.

frying Salt to taste

Directions:

1. Salt the water and add the flour.
2. Make a few openings in the focal point of the mixture and pour warm explained butter.
3. Knead the batter and let represent 15 minutes, covered.
4. Shape into six balls.
5. Flatten the balls into six slight rounds utilizing a rolling pin.
6. Heat sufficient oil to cover a round griddle completely.
7. Place a puri in it when hot.
8. Fry for 20 seconds on each side.
9. Place on a paper towel.
10. Repeat with the remainder of the puri and serve.

Nutrition:

.

Calories: 106

.

Fat: 3 g

.

Carb: 6 g

.

Protein: 3 g

100. Pita Bread

Preparation Time: 10 minutes Cooking Time: 15 minutes
Servings: 8
Ingredients:

2 cups almond flour, sifted

½ cup of water

2 tbsp. olive oil

Salt, to taste

1 tbsp. black cumin

Directions:

1. Preheat the stove to 400 0F.
2. Combine the flour with salt. Add the water and olive oil.
3. Knead the batter and let represent around 15 minutes.
4. Shape the batter into eight balls.
5. Line a baking sheet with material paper and smooth the balls into eight flimsy rounds.
6. Sprinkle dark cumin.
7. Bake for 15 minutes, serve.

Nutrition:

Calories: 73

.

Fat: 6.9 g

.

Carbohydrates: 1.6 g

.

Protein: 1.6 g

101. Almond Flour Apple Bread Rolls

Preparation Time: 10 minutes
 Cooking Time: 30 minutes
Servings: 6
Ingredients:

.

1 cup boiling water or as needed

.

2 cups almond flour

.

½ cup ground flaxseed

- 4 tbsp. Psyllium husk powder

- 1 tbsp. Baking powder

- 2 tbsp. Olive oil

- 2 eggs

- 1 tbsp. apple cider vinegar

- ½ tbsp. of salt

Directions

1. Preheat the broiler to 350 0F.
2. In a bowl, combine as one the almond flour, baking powder, psyllium husk powder, flaxseed flour, and salt.
3. Add the olive oil and eggs and mix until the combination takes after breadcrumbs, then, at that point, blend in the apple juice vinegar.
4. Slowly add bubbling water and blend it into the combination. Let represent thirty minutes to firm up.
5. Line material paper over the baking tray.
6. Using your hands, make a bundle of the dough.
7. Transfer mixture balls on a baking plate and heat for 30 minutes, or until firm and golden.

Nutrition:

.

Calories: 301

.

Fat: 24.1 g

.

Carb: 5 g

.

Protein: 11 g

102. Low Carb Bread

Preparation Time: 10 minutes
 Cooking Time: 21 minutes
 Servings: 12
Ingredients:

-

- 2 cups mozzarella cheese,

- grated 8 oz. cream cheese

- Herbs and spices to taste

- 1 tbsp. baking powder

- 1 cup crushed pork rinds

- ¼ cup parmesan cheese, grated

-

3 large eggs

Directions

1. Preheat broiler to 375 0F.
2. Line material paper over the baking pan.
3. In a bowl, place cream cheddar and mozzarella and microwave for 1 moment on high power. Mix and microwave for brief more. Then, at that point, mix again.
4. Stir in egg parmesan, pork skins, spices, flavors, and baking powder until mixed.
5. Spread blend on the baking dish and heat until the top is daintily brown around 15 to 20 minutes.
6. Cool, cut, and serve.

Nutrition:

.

Calories: 166

.

Fat: 13 g

.

Carb: 1 g

.

Protein: 9 g

103. Splendid Low-Carb Bread

Preparation Time: 15 minutes
Cooking Time: 60 to 70 minutes
Servings: 12
Ingredients:

.

½ tbsp. Herbs, such as basil, rosemary, or oregano

.

½ tbsp. Garlic or onion powder

.

1 tbsp. Baking powder

.

5 tbsp. Psyllium husk powder

.

½ cup almond flour

.

½ cup coconut flour

.

¼ tbsp. Salt

·

1 ½ cup egg whites

·

3 tbsp. Oil or melted butter

·

2 tbsp. Apple cider vinegar

·

1/3 to ¾ cup hot water

Directions

1. Grease a portion container and preheat the stove to 350 0F.
2. In a bowl, whisk the salt, psyllium husk powder, onion or garlic powder, coconut flour, almond flour, and baking powder.
3. Stir in egg whites, oil, and apple juice vinegar. One small step at a time add the heated water, mixing until batter expansion in size. Try not to add an excess of water.
4. Mold the mixture into a square shape and move to an oil portion pan.
5. Bake in the broiler for 60 to 70 minutes, or until outside layer feels firm and brown on top.
6. Cool and serve.

Nutrition:

·

Calories: 97

.

Fat: 5.7 g

.

Carb: 7.5 g

.

Protein: 4.1 g

104. Bread Machine Country White Bread

Preparation Time: 10 minutes
Cooking Time: 2 hours
Servings: 1 Loaf
Ingredients:

.

1 1/2 cups of water, lukewarm

.

2 1/2 cups of all-purpose flour

.

1 cup of bread flour

- 1/4 tsp. of baking soda

- 2 1/2 tsp. of a bread machine or instant yeast

- 1 tbsp. plus one tsp. of olive oil

- 1 1/2 tsp. of sugar

- 1 tsp. of salt

Directions:

1. In the arrangement proposed by your bread machine organization, add every one of the fixings to your bread machine pan.
2. Use the medium covering and the fast or moderate setting press start.
3. Turn the bread out to cool onto a shelf.
4. Cut, and have fun!

Nutrition:

- Calories: 319

- Fats 5.6 g

- Carbohydrates 3 g

- Protein: 9.6 g

CHAPTER 10:

Sweet, Chocolate and Fruit Bread

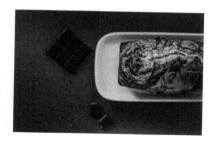

105. Blueberry Bread

Preparation Time: 3 hours 15 minutes
Cooking Time: 40-45 minutes
Servings: 1 loaf
Ingredients:

.

$1^1/8$ to 1¼ cups water

.

6 ounces cream cheese, softened

.

2 tbsp. butter or margarine

.

¼ cup of sugar

.

2 tsp. salt

.

4½ cups bread flour

.

1½ tsp. grated lemon peel

.

2 tsp. cardamom

.

2 tbsp. nonfat: dry milk

.

2½ tsp. red star brand active dry yeast

.

²/3 cup dried blueberries

Directions:

1. Place all fixings aside from dried blueberries in the bread dish, utilizing minimal measure of fluid recorded in the formula. Select the light outside setting and raisin/nut cycle. Press start.

2. Observe the batter as it works. Following 5 to 10 minutes, assuming it seems dry and solid or on the other hand on the off chance that your machine seems as though it's stressing to ply it, add more fluid 1 tbsp. at a time until dough shapes a smooth, delicate, flexible ball that is marginally crude to the touch.

3. At the blare, add the dried blueberries.
 4. After the baking cycle closes, eliminate bread from the container, place on cake rack, and permit to cool 1 hour before slicing.

Nutrition:

·

Calories: 180

·

Fat: 3 g

·

Carbohydrate: 250 g

·

Protein: 9 g

106. Date Delight Bread

Preparation Time: 2 hours
Cooking Time: 15 minutes
Servings: 12
Ingredients:

.

¾ cup water, lukewarm

.

½ cup milk, lukewarm

.

1 tbsp. butter, melted at room temperature

.

¼ cup honey

.

1 tbsp. molasses

.

1 tbsp. sugar

.

¼ cups whole-wheat flour

.

1 ¼ cups white bread

.

flour 1 tbsp. skim milk

.

powder 1 tsp. salt

.

1 tbsp. unsweetened cocoa powder

.

1 ½ tsp. instant or bread machine yeast

.

¾ cup chopped dates

Directions:

1. Take 1 ½ pound size portion dish and first add the fluid fixings and afterward add the dry fixings. (Try not to add the dates as of now.)

2. Place the portion dish in the machine and close its top lid.

3. Plug the bread machine into a power attachment. For choosing a bread cycle, press "Fundamental bread/white bread/standard bread" or "Organic product/nut bread" and for choosing a hull type, press "light" or "medium."

4. Start the machine and it will begin setting up the bread. At the point when the machine blares or transmissions, add the dates.

5. After the bread portion is finished, open the top and take out the portion pan.

6. Allow the skillet to chill off for 10-15 minutes on a wire rack. Delicately shake the skillet and eliminate the bread loaf.

7. Make cuts and serve.

Nutrition:

.

Calories: 220

.

Fat: 5 g

.

Carbohydrate: 52 g

.

Protein: 4 g

107. Blueberry Honey Bread

Preparation Time: 2 hours
Cooking Time: 15 minutes
Servings: 12
Ingredients:

- ¾ cup milk, lukewarm

- 1 egg at room temperature

- ¼ tbsp. butter, melted at room temperature

- 1 ½ tbsp. honey

- ½ cup rolled oats

- ⅓ cups white bread flour

- 1 ⅛ tsp. salt

- 1 ½ tsp. instant or bread machine yeast

½ cup dried blueberries

Directions:

1. Take 1 ½ pound size portion dish and first add the fluid fixings and afterward add the dry fixings. (Try not to add the blueberries as of now.)

2. Place the portion container in the machine and close its top lid.
3. Plug the bread machine into a power attachment. For choosing a bread cycle, press "Essential bread/white bread/customary bread" or "Natural product/nut bread" and for choosing a covering type, press "Light" or "Medium."
4. Start the machine and it will begin setting up the bread. At the point when the machine blares or transmissions, add the blueberries.
5. After the bread portion is finished, open the top and take out the portion pan.
6. Allow the container to chill off for 10-15 minutes on a wire rack. Delicately shake the container and eliminate the bread loaf.
7. Make cuts and serve.

Nutrition:

Calories: 180

Fat: 3 g

Carbohydrate: 250 g

Protein: 9 g

108. Orange and Walnut Bread

Preparation Time: 2 hours 50 minutes
 Cooking Time: 45 minutes
 Servings: 10-15
 Ingredients:

.

1 egg white

.

1 tbsp. water

.

½ cup warm

.

whey 1 tbsp.
 yeast

.

4 tbsp. sugar

.

2 oranges, crushed

.

4 cups flour

.

1 tsp. salt

.

1 and ½ tbsp.

.

salt 3 tsp. orange

.

peel 1/3 tsp.
 vanilla

.

3 tbsp. walnut and almonds, crushed

.

1 tsp. Crushed pepper, salt, cheese for garnish

Directions:

1. Add every one of the fixings to your Bread Machine (aside from egg white, 1 tbsp. water, and squashed pepper/cheese).
2. Set the program to"Batter" cycle and let the cycle run.
3. Remove the mixture (utilizing gently floured hands) and cautiously place it on a floured surface.
4. Cover with a light film/stick paper and let the mixture ascend for 10 minutes.
5. Divide the batter into thirds after it has risen
6. Place on a daintily flour surface, fold each piece into 14x10 inches estimated rectangles
7. Use a sharp blade to cut painstakingly cut the batter into strips of½ inch width
8. Pick 2-3 strips and turn them on numerous occasions, making a point to press the closures together
9. Preheat your stove to 400 °F
10. Take a bowl and mix egg white, water, and brush onto the breadsticks
11. Sprinkle salt, pepper/cheese
12. Bake for 10-12 minutes until brilliant brown
13. Remove from baking sheet and move to cooling rack Serve and enjoy!

Nutrition:

.

Calories: 437

.

Fat: 7 g

.

Carbohydrate: 82 g

.

Protein: 12 g

109. Lemon and Poppy Buns

Preparation Time: 2 hours 50 minutes
 Cooking Time: 45 minutes
 Servings: 10-20 buns
 Ingredients:

.

1 tbsp. melted butter for grease

.

1 and 1/3 cups hot water

.

3 tbsp. powdered milk

.

2 tbsp. Crisco shortening

.

1 and ½ tsp. salt

.

1 tbsp. lemon juice

.

4 and ¼ cups bread flour

.

½ tsp. nutmeg

.

2 tsp. grated lemon rind

.

2 tbsp. poppy seeds

.

1 and ¼ tsp. yeast

.

2 tsp. wheat gluten

Directions:

1. Add each of the fixings to your Bread Machine (aside from dissolved butter).
2. Set the program to "Mixture" cycle and let the cycle run.
3. Remove the batter (utilizing daintily floured hands) and cautiously place it on a floured surface.
4. Cover with a light film/stick paper and let the mixture ascend for 10 minutes.
5. Take a huge treat sheet and oil it with butter.
6. Cut the risen mixture into 15-20 pieces and shape them into balls.
7. Place the balls onto the sheet (2 inches separated) and cover.
8. Place in a warm spot and allowed them to ascend for 30-40 minutes until the batter doubles.
9. Preheat your broiler to 375 °F, move the treat sheet to your broiler and heat for 12-15 minutes. Brush the top with a bit of margarine, enjoy!

Nutrition:
.Calories: 231 .

Fat: 11 g

Carbohydrate: 31 g

Protein: 4 g

110. Chocolate Chip Peanut Butter Banana Bread

Preparation Time: 25 minutes
Cooking Time: 10 minutes
Servings: 12 to 16 cuts
Ingredients:

2 bananas, mashed

.

2 eggs, at room temperature

.

1/2 cup melted butter, cooled

.

2 tbsp. milk, at room temperature

.

1 tsp. pure vanilla extract

.

2 cups all-purpose flour

.

1/2 cup sugar

.

11/4 tsp. baking powder

.

1/2 tsp. baking soda

.

1/2 tsp. salt

.

1/2 cup peanut butter chips

.

1/2 cup semisweet chocolate chips

Directions:

1. Stir together the bananas, eggs, spread, milk, and vanilla in the bread machine container and set it aside.
2. In a medium bowl, throw together the flour, sugar, baking powder, baking pop, salt, peanut butter chips, and chocolate chips.
3. Add the dry fixings to the bucket.
4. Program the machine for speedy/fast bread, and press start.
5. When the cake is made, stick a blade into it, and assuming that it emerges out perfect, the portion is done.
6. If the portion needs a couple of more minutes, take a gander at the administration board for a heat possibly button, and expand the time by 10 minutes.
9. Gently rock the can to eliminate the bread and turn it out onto a rack to cool.

Nutrition:

.

Calories: 297

.

Fat: 14 g

Carbohydrates: 40 g

Protein: 4 g

111. Chocolate Sour Cream Bread

Preparation Time: 25 minutes
Cooking Time: 10 minutes
Servings: 12 cuts Ingredients:

.

1 cup sour cream

.

2 eggs, at room

.

temperature 1 cup of sugar

.

1/2 cup (1 stick) butter, at room temperature

- 1/4 cup plain Greek yogurt

- 13/4 cups all-purpose flour

- 1/2 cup unsweetened cocoa powder

- 1/2 tsp. baking powder

- 1/2 tsp. salt

- 1 cup milk chocolate chips

Directions:

1. In a little bowl, stay together the harsh cream, eggs, sugar, spread, and yogurt until just combined.
2. Transfer the wet fixings to the bread machine pail, and afterward add the flour, cocoa powder, baking powder, salt, and chocolate chips.
3. Program the machine for speedy/quick bread, and press start.
4. When the portion is done, stick a blade into it, and in the event that it tells the truth, the portion is done.
5. If the portion needs a couple of more minutes, check the control board for a prepare possibly button and broaden the time by 10 minutes.

8.
.Gently rock the can to eliminate the portion and spot it out onto a rack to cool.

Nutrition:
Calories: 347

.

Fat: 16 g

.

Carbohydrates: 48 g

.

Protein: 6 g

112. Brownie Bread

Preparation Time: 1 hour 15 minutes
Cooking Time: 50 minutes
Servings: 1 portion
Ingredients:

- 1 egg

- 1 egg yolk

- 1 tsp. salt

- 1/2 cup boiling water

- 1/2 cup cocoa powder, unsweetened

- 1/2 cup warm water

- 2 1/2 tsp. Active dry

- yeast 2 tbsp. Vegetable oil

- 2 tsp. White sugar

- 2/3 cup white sugar

- 3 cups bread flour

Directions:

1. Put the cocoa powder in a little bow. Pour bubbling water and disintegrate the cocoa powder.
2. Put the warm water, yeast, and the two tsp. White sugar in another bowl. Disintegrate yeast and sugar. Let represent around 10 minutes, or until the blend is creamy.
3. Place the cocoa blend, the yeast blend, the flour, the 2/3 cup white sugar, the salt, the vegetable, and the egg in the bread skillet. Select essential bread cycle. Press start.

Nutrition:

- Calories: 70

- Fat: 3 g

- Carbohydrates: 10 g

Protein: 1 g

113. Black Forest Bread

Preparation Time: 2 hours 15 minutes
 Cooking Time: 50 minutes
 Servings: 1 portion
 Ingredients:

.

1 1/8 cups warm water

.

1/3 cup molasses

.

1 1/2 tbsp. canola oil

.

1 1/2 cups bread flour

.

1 cup Rye flour

.

1 cup whole wheat flour

.

1 1/2 tsp. salt

.

3 tbsp. cocoa powder

.

1 1/2 tbsp. caraway seeds

.

2 tsp. active dry yeast

Directions:

1. Place all ingredients into your bread maker according to manufacture.
2. Select sort to a light hull, then, at that point, press start.
3. If the combination is excessively dry, add a tbsp. of warm water at a time.
4. If the blend is excessively wet, add flour again a little at a time.
5. The combination ought to go into a ball structure, and simply delicate and somewhat tacky to the finger contact. It goes for a wide range of bread when kneading.

Nutrition:

.

Calories: 240

.

Fat: 4 g

.

Carbohydrates: 29 g

.

Protein: 22 g

---

114. Honey Sourdough Bread

Preparation Time: 15 minutes; multi week (Starter) Cooking Time: 3 hours
Servings: 1 portion
Ingredients:

.

2/3 cup sourdough starter

.

1/2 cup water

.

1 tbsp. vegetable oil

.

2 tbsp. honey

1/2 tsp. salt

1/2 cup high Protein: wheat flour

2 cups bread flour

1 tsp. active dry yeast

Directions:

1. Measure 1 cup of starter and remaining bread fixings, add to bread machine pan.
2. Choose essential/white bread cycle with medium or light outside layer color.

Nutrition:

Calories: 175

Fat: 0.3 g

Carbohydrate: 33 g

.

Protein: 5.6 g

115. Sweet Almond Anise Bread

Preparation Time: 2 hours 20 minutes
 Cooking Time: 50 minutes
 Servings: 1 portion
 Ingredients:

.

3/4 cup water

.

1/4 cup

.

butter 1/4

.

cup sugar 1/2
 tsp. salt

.

3 cups bread flour

.

1 tsp. anise seed

.

2 tsp. active dry yeast

.

1/2 cup almonds, chopped

Directions:

1. Add each of the fixings to your bread machine, cautiously adhering to the guidelines of the manufacturer.
2. Choose the arrangement of your bread machine to fundamental/white bread and set hull type to medium.
3. Press start.
4. Wait until the cycle completes.
5. Once the portion is prepared, take the can out and afterward permit the portion to cool for 5 minutes.
6. Gently shake the pail to eliminate the loaf.
7. Transfer to a cooling rack, cut, and serve.
8. Enjoy!

Nutrition:

.

Calories: 87

.

Fat: 4 g

.

Carbohydrates: 7 g

.

Protein: 3 g

116. Chocolate Ginger and Hazelnut Bread

Preparation Time: 2 hours 50 minutes
Cooking Time: 45 minutes
Servings: 2 portions
Ingredients:

.

1/2 cup chopped hazelnuts

.

2 tsp. bread machine yeast

.

3 1/2 cups bread flour

.

1 tsp. salt

.

1 1/2 tbsp. dry skim milk powder

.

3 tbsp. light brown sugar

.

2 tbsp. candied ginger, chopped

.

1/3 cup unsweetened coconut

.

1 1/2 tbsp. unsalted butter, cubed

.

1 cup, plus two tbsp. water, with a temperature of 80 to 90 °F(26 to 32 °C)

Directions:

1. Put every one of the fixings, aside from the hazelnuts, in the dish in a specific order: water, spread, coconut, candy-coated ginger, earthy colored sugar, milk, salt, flour, and yeast.

2. Secure the container in the machine and close the cover. Put the toasted hazelnuts in the leafy foods dispenser.

 3. Turn the machine on. Select the essential setting and your ideal shade of the covering and press start.

 4. Once done, cautiously move the heated bread to a wire rack until cooled.

Nutrition:

.

Calories: 273

.

Fat: 11 g

.

Carbohydrate: 43 g

.

Protein: 7 g

117. White Chocolate Bread

Preparation Time: 3 hours
 Cooking Time: 15 minutes
 Servings: 12
 Ingredients:

.

1/4 cup warm water

- 1 cup warm milk

- 1 egg

- 1/4 cup butter, softened

- 3 cups bread flour

- 2 tbsp. brown

- sugar 2 tbsp. white
sugar 1 tsp. salt

- 1 tsp. ground cinnamon

- 1 (.25 oz.) package active dry yeast

1 cup white chocolate chips

Directions:

1. Put every one of the fixings together, aside from the white chocolate chips, into the bread machine pan.
2. Choose the cycle on the machine and press the beginning button to run the machine.
3. Put in the white chocolate chips at the machine's transmission assuming the gadget utilized has a natural product setting on it, or you might set the white chocolate chips around 5 minutes before the massaging cycle ends.

Nutrition:

.

Calories: 277

.

Fat: 10.5 g

.

Carbohydrate: 39 g

.

Protein: 6.6 g

118. Chocolate Chip Bread

Preparation Time: 10 minutes
 Cooking Time: 2 hours 50 minutes
 Servings: 1 loaf
 Ingredients:

·

1/4 cup water 1

·

cup milk

·

1 egg

·

3 cups bread flour 3

·

tbsp. brown sugar 2

·

tbsp. white sugar 1

·

tsp. salt

.

1 tsp. ground cinnamon

.

1 1/2 tsp. active dry yeast 2

.

tbsp. margarine, softened

.

3/4 cup semisweet chocolate chips 1. Add every one of the fixings into the container with the exception of chocolate chips.
2. Choose blend bread
3. When the machine signals, add in chips.

Nutrition:

.

Calories: 184

.

Fat: 5.2 g

.

Carbohydrate: 30.6 g

.

Protein: 3.5 g

---

119. Peanut Butter Bread

Preparation Time: 10 minutes
Cooking Time: 3 hours
Servings: 1 loaf
Ingredients:

.

1 1/4 cups water

.

1/2 cup peanut butter - creamy or chunky 1

.

1/2 cups whole wheat flour

.

3 tbsp. gluten flour

.

1 1/2 cups bread flour

- 1/4 cup brown sugar 1/2

- tsp. salt

- 2 1/4 tsp. active dry yeast

Directions:
1. Add every one of the fixings into the pan. 2. Choose entire wheat bread setting huge loaf.

Nutrition:

- Calories: 82

- Fat: 2.2 g

- Carbohydrate: 13 g

- Protein: 2.5 g

120. Jam Rolls

Preparation Time: 10 minutes
Cooking Time: 40 minutes
Servings: 12
Ingredients:
Dough:

.1 cup warm milk

.

0 3 cup butter

.

0 5 cup granulated sugar 2 somewhat

.

beaten eggs

.

1 2 tsp salt

.

4 cups bread flour

.

1 tsp . dynamic dry yeast
Filling:

0 5 cup relaxed butter

0 5 cup blended great quality jam **Topping:**

0.5 cup melted and cooled to room temperature butter Granulated sugar for sprinkling

1. Warm the milk in the microwave for forty seconds.
2. Place milk dissolved margarine and sugar in the bread machine and

stir.
3. Let sit for 20 minutes.
4. Stir in salt and the eggs.
5. Add flour and spot yeast on top of the flour.
6. Select the mixture cycle.
7. Start the machine.
8. Butter a baking skillet and set aside.
9. Roll batter into a rectangle.
10. Spread with spread then with jam.
11. Roll up to make a long log and cut it in half.
12. Slice each piece in half again and cut every one of the quarters into 3 slices.
13. Place rolls in the pan.
14. Brush with softened butter.
15. Sprinkle with sugar.
16. Cover with plastic wrap.
17. Let ascend for thirty minutes.
18. Preheat the broiler to 400 °F.
19. Bake for 18 minutes until brilliant brown.
20. Let them cool completely.

Nutrition: .

Calories: 230

- Fat: 5 g

- Carbohydrates: 38 g

- Protein: 26 g

APPENDIX: CONVERSION TABLES

US Dry Volume Measurements

1/16 tsp. a dash
1/8 tsp. a pinch
3 tsp. 1 tbsp.
¼ cup 4 tbsp.
1/3 cup 5 tbsp. + 1 tsp. ½ cup 8 tbsp.
¾ cup 12 tbsp.
1 cup 16 tbsp.
1 pound 16 ounces

US Liquid Volume Measurements

Eight fluid ounces 1 cup
1 pint = 2 cups 16 fluid ounces
1 quart = 2 pints 4 cups
1 gallon = 4 quarts 16 cups

CONCLUSION

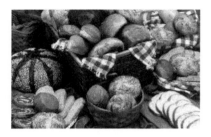

Depending on what sort of home cook you are, bread is either an absolute necessity know transitional experience or a scary objective you haven't exactly gathered the mental fortitude to attempt. This is on the grounds that bread is a work serious food where slight slip-ups can immensely affect the eventual outcome. A large portion of us depend on locally acquired bread, yet whenever you've tasted custom made bread, it's enticing to make your own as regularly as could really be expected. A bread machine makes the interaction easier.

Making a portion of bread feels like a significant achievement. Why? There are a ton of steps. Blending manipulating sealing resting forming lastly baking.

You know how to make bread the hard way, so how does the bread-making machine get it done? A bread machine is essentially a little, electric stove. It fits one enormous bread tin with an extraordinary hub associated with the electric engine. A metal oar associates with the pivot, and this massages the batter. Assuming you were making the bread in a blender, you would most likely utilize a batter snare, and in certain directions, you'll see the bread machine's plying part alluded to as a snare or "blades."

The first thing you do is take out the tin and add the bread dough you made in Step 1. Bread machines can make any kind of bread, whether it's made from normal white flour, whole wheat, etc. Pop this tin into the axle and program by selecting the type of bread, which includes options like basic, wholewheat, multigrain, and so on. There are even cycles specifically for sweetbread; bread with nuts, seeds, and raisins; gluten-free; and bagels. Many models also let you cook jam.

You'll presumably see a"mixture" mode choice, as well. You would involve that one for pizza. The machine doesn't really cook anything it simply plies and afterward you take out the pizza batter and prepare it in your ordinary broiler. On the off chance that you're not making pizza mixture, the following determinations you'll make are the portion size and hull type. Whenever those are picked, press the "clock" button. In view of your different determinations, a period will appear and you should simply push "start."

After manipulating and before the machine starts baking many individuals will eliminate the batter so they can take out the working oars since they regularly make an indent in the completed bread. The oars ought to just jump out or you can purchase an exceptional snare that makes the evacuation simpler. Presently you can return the bread to the machine. The top is shut during the baking system. In the event that it's a glass top, you can really see what's happening. You'll hear the oar turning on the engine, plying the mixture. It lies still for the rising stage and afterward begins again for seriously manipulating if essential. The engine is additionally off for the demonstrating stage. Then, the warming component turns on, and steam ascends from the exhaust vent as the bread prepares. The entire cycle typically takes a couple hours.

There's a ton of work engaged with making bread manually. At the point when you utilize a machine, that machine does a ton of the bustling stuff for you. You simply place your mixture and the bread producer begins doing its thing giving you an opportunity to do different errands or take a load off. As a note, not all bread creators are totally programmed, so assuming you need this advantage, maybe you'll need to pay somewhat more cash. However, it's worth the effort for a many individuals.

Lightning Source UK Ltd.
Milton Keynes UK
UKHW050815040422
401060UK00005B/106

9 781804 340639